```
920              192533
D74t             10.95
Dossick

Transplant: a family chronicle
```

| DATE DUE | | | |
|---|---|---|---|
| MR 26 '90 | | | |
| MR 5 '92 | | | |
| | | | |
| | | | |
| | | | |
| | | | |
| | | | |
| | | | |
| | | | |
| | | | |
| | | | |
| | | | |

ST. CLOUD PUBLIC LIBRARY
**GREAT RIVER REGIONAL LIBRARY**
St. Cloud, Minnesota  56301

# TRANSPLANT

# TRANSPLANT
## *A Family Chronicle*

---

PHILIP DOSSICK

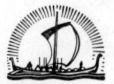

THE VIKING PRESS
NEW YORK

Copyright © Philip Dossick, 1978
All rights reserved

First published in 1978 by The Viking Press
625 Madison Avenue, New York, N.Y. 10022
Published simultaneously in Canada by
Penguin Books Canada Limited

LIBRARY OF CONGRESS CATALOGING IN PUBLICATION DATA
Dossick, Philip.
  Transplant.

  1. Heart—Transplant—Biography.
2. Dossick, Philip. I. Title.
RD598.D62      362.1′9′7412 [B]      77-27290
ISBN 0-670-72427-0

Printed in the United States of America

Set in Computer Times Roman

for Jane

*First*

He is the strongest man I have ever known.
And the most courageous.
She is the bravest woman I have ever known.
And the most gentle.

# *An Appreciation*

This is a true story.

Let me tell you how I came to write it.

A couple of years ago, I read about John Hurley in one of the papers. I thought it might be interesting to write about him, so I sent him a note. About a month later, he called and invited me out to his place.

I drove out (it's a half a tank of gas from New York), and found one of the most exasperating, stubborn, iron-willed, racist, chauvinistic, and finally heroic men I've ever known.

A powerhouse.

He poured me a bourbon and water and started to seduce me. *Told* me I was going to write about him. Fifteen minutes later, he had me believing him.

First, he showed me his scars (and there are many). Then he told me the crudest, the filthiest, the most scabrous joke I have ever heard in my life. I was at once appalled and fascinated.

He introduced me to his wife, Ann. She was, of course, his

polar opposite. Sensitive, graceful, a little shy. With an undercurrent of stability, strength, and quiet dignity.

I asked him to tell me a little bit about his background, and he did, while Ann brought out the Devil Dogs.

John Hurley is a former Brooklyn slum kid who worked his way up out of Park Slope the hard way. Trade school. Navy. Night school.

By the time he was thirty-five, he and Ann were living in an exclusive suburb of New Jersey, with their three children. And his hunting dog.

He had become a divisional director of Sea-Land Service, Inc., directly responsible for coordinating their mammoth fleet of refrigerated trailer trucks, the largest shipping fleet of its kind in the world.

Then he was stricken with a catastrophic heart attack.

For openers.

He caught me staring at the scars on his chest. And he knew exactly what was on my mind. So he answered my first question before I had a chance to ask it.

"Phil, until after the operation, I didn't know if I was getting the heart of a wop or a woman, black or white, Oriental or Hebrew. And frankly, I didn't give a damn."

And this book was born.

We began our conversations. Hundreds of them.

What follows, told entirely in their own words, are the self-portraits of two Americans, John and Ann Hurley, including their memories and their impressions of themselves as they seek to cope with the most terrifying chapter of their lives.

PHILIP DOSSICK

*Sierra Mews*
*Ipswich, Massachusetts*
*May 1, 1977*

# *Conversations*

## August 1975—August 1976

Usually held across the kitchen table, a favorite spot before the children came home from school, with kosher salami sandwiches and beer. Also in the back yard; during walks through Byram Township, Forest Lakes; in the Municipal Building, Eskil's office; over cards with the Tamarack Inn regulars, for whom bartenders Willy and Jack do sensitive service; in Hahn's bakery (for brownies), the Sussex and Merchants Midlantic Bank, the Sheer Happiness Beauty Salon, Les's American Hardware Store, Perona Farms, Grist Mill Shopping Plaza, Mountainside Diner, Lenape Valley Regional High School, the Cranberry Lake Fire Department, Adam Todd Inn, Vinnie's Texaco Station, Roxbury Medical Center, Andover A&P, Violet Johnson's The Scandinavian Shop, Dempsey's Liquor Store, Turner's Wine Cellar, Wagner's Bait and Tackle, The Big "N" in Newton, Sam Palumbo's Barber Shop, County College of Morris, Melody Dance School, Britt's Department Store, Andover Pharmacy, Tamarack Delicatessen, Economy Department Store, Faith Baptist Kindergarten, Town and Country Deli on U.S. 206, Sears Roebuck and Co., Sea-Land headquarters, and the downstairs bedroom.

# Contents

**ONE:** THE SCENE OF AN ACCIDENT
1. *Heart Attack* 3
2. *Home* 19
3. *No Hope* 27
4. *The Two of Us* 32
5. *The Secret* 48
6. *Out* 54
7. *Fear, Money, and Anger* 57
8. *The Childhood Years* 62
9. *Dying* 71

**TWO:** TRANSPLANT
10. *Orders* 93
11. *Stanford University Medical Center* 103
12. *Psychological Tests* 113

13. *Yes*   130
14. *And Counting*   143
15. *The Surgery*   153
16. *The Vigil*   159
17. *Hurley Power*   170
18. *The First Acute Rejection*   174
19. *Out of the Hospital*   183
20. *Anchored to the Clinic*   193
21. *Janice*   204
22. *Rest and Relaxation*   215

THREE: A TRUCE WITH TIME
23. *Return Ticket*   229
24. *Recovery at Home*   236
25. *The Second Acute Rejection*   248
26. *A New Life*   258
27. *Champagne*   267

AUTHOR'S NOTE   272
DEDICATION   273
ACKNOWLEDGMENTS   274

# ONE

## THE SCENE OF AN ACCIDENT

# 1

## Heart Attack

***JOHN*** I was thirty-five years old.

And I was out on the lawn, weeding the garden.

This was April 19, 1971. A Saturday.

We live in a private, lakefront community called Forest Lakes. It's very secluded. Our house was built for us, from an architect's plans. In a contemporary design. We've furnished it in Early American style. It's big.

The mumps were going around the lake. I started getting this tightening in my neck—you know, like you have a swollen gland? This is the way I had it, on both sides of my neck. And I said to Ann, "Jeez, I hope I'm not getting the mumps." So then I had a couple of beers and a cheese sandwich, and it went away.

That night we went down to the drive-in. We saw *Patton*. Then we came home and went to bed. I was awakened out of a sound sleep really, and I had these tremendous chest pains. And my shoulders, and again my neck. I could feel this almost lump in my neck. So I asked Ann to get me some Pepto-Bismol.

None of our friends had ever had heart attacks. You just don't think about something like that. I was thirty-five. It was inconceivable. You just think it's indigestion. So I took the Pepto-Bismol, and in about a half hour or so, the pain was gone. The two of us went back to sleep.

A short time later—again I came out of a dead sleep. That same thing. And this time I had a problem breathing. Hard to breathe. So I opened the sliding glass doors that face out on the back yard, and let the air in. The air hits me—and I break out into a cold sweat. The pain is centered right smack in the middle of my chest. And I felt nauseous. Sick.

I took some more Pepto-Bismol. That's when Ann wanted to call the ambulance. She didn't think it was a heart attack, but that I might have food poisoning of some kind.

I slept sitting up in my smoking chair the whole night.

When I woke up Sunday morning, I felt fine again. Pains were gone. I felt great. Like it never happened. As a matter of fact, I even helped prepare dinner. My boss from Sea-Land was over, Jim Clark, and his wife Jean.

We had a barbecue. Jim and I, we barbecued outside. Steaks. Char-broiled and *sizzling*.

After the barbecue, we're sitting in the dining room, drinking Black Russians on the rocks. Jim's specialty. Vodka and Kahlua. We finished off God knows how many of 'em. And after a while we were feeling pretty mellow. Jean had to drive them home.

But that Sunday I felt one hundred percent.

Monday morning I'm sitting in the kitchen, at breakfast. There's a mad rush on, with the baby, John Jr., being fed, little one-year-old Joanie toddling around, and Janice, the teen-ager, getting ready for school, and Ann asks me how I feel, because I guess I had a funny look on my face. She asks me, "Do you have any pain again? Or indigestion?" And I say, "I don't know what it is. But would you listen to my chest? I feel a kind of fluttering inside."

So she comes over—she's not the greatest in the morning—and by this time, with the kids shouting and throwing cereal and messing the joint up, she's had it, and she comes over and listens to my chest, puts her ear right up against it and says, "Oh yeah, John. I think I hear something. It's going *thump thump thump thump!*"

So I say, "Kiss my ass!" and walk out the door for work, and slam it shut behind me.

I did feel kinda funny inside. Like my heart was missing beats or something. Palpitations. But with the confusion with the children, and I'd been drunk the night before, I thought I was just hung over.

So I drove in to work. And as I'm going toward my office I'm thinking, Gee, you know about these mumps. I hope I'm not getting the mumps! Because I felt . . . *strange.* Just very strange. There was this sort of *tightening* in my neck.

Ed Coonan comes over to me. He's a VP in charge of the Caribbean operations, and he says, "John, tomorrow there's a very important meeting been scheduled. We think we can corner the cocoa market coming up from Santo Domingo! There's *millions* involved!"

"Great. Beautiful."

"The meeting's in Santo Domingo. Can you pack a toothbrush and fly down with me tomorrow? We've got to meet with the exporters. This is a big one, John. And I can taste it."

I said sure.

But at the same time I'm thinking about these mumps. I figure, Jeez, if I go down to Santo Domingo and I get sick down there, what in the hell's gonna happen? Santo Domingo is no place for *mumps.*

So I call home and I ask Ann—I had no family physician at that time, I'd never really been sick a day in my life—so I ask Ann to get me an appointment with a doctor because I've got to go to Santo Domingo on a nine o'clock flight in the morning.

She calls the Roxbury Medical Center. There are no openings in anybody's schedule. She tells them that I had had severe chest pains two days prior, and that I was about to travel out of the country on a business trip to the Caribbean, and we thought it a good idea if I have an examination. Just to be on the safe side. They gave me an appointment for 3:00 that afternoon. Come 1:00, I left work.

If you're at all familiar with New Jersey, Route 22 is the worst road to be on in the state. Slow as bee honey. Absolutely unreal. It crawls. So I'm on 22, when all of a sudden I just feel—*BOOM!* Something is *exploding* in my chest. The same type of a thing I had on Saturday night. Only *much* worse. And my hands are *frozen* to the wheel. And I'm saying to myself *it'll let up, it'll let up, it'll let up, it's gotta let up!* But instead of letting up, it's getting worse and worse, and it's getting worse still!

Now mind you, *I've got seventy more miles to drive.* So I'm driving and driving and thank God *I'm going to the doctor!* And I'm saying to myself, Holy jeez, maybe this *is* a heart attack! But what in hell am I gonna do? I'm on Route 22! Am I just gonna pull off the road and try to find some *strange* doctor?

Really. What do you do? I knew I had the appointment with this doctor at the medical center. If I got to him. At least he was there waiting for me. So I drove to the center as fast as I could. Took almost an hour and a half. I pull into the parking lot, look at my watch, and I'm forty-five minutes early for the appointment!

I know doctors are very prompt. Very strict about time. So I'm sitting in the waiting area, and the pain is getting worse and worse. Like a clamp pressing on my chest, crushing me. And I'm sitting there, swallowing, sweating, and *pulling* the air in. A half hour goes by. It's getting unbearable. I go to the phone booth and call Ann.

"I'm not staying here any more."

"Why not? What's the matter?"

"Ann, I'm in severe pain—and they're not taking me!"

"Did you tell the nurse?"

"No."

So she starts yelling at me. "Get over there to that goddamn nurse and tell her that you need medical attention immediately!"

"No. I can't do that."

"Go and tell them you need a doctor."

"It's not my turn yet. I'm still fifteen minutes early."

So she gets hysterical. "That's a typical man for you! A woman would get up and go over to the nurse and say, 'I'm in severe pain. Can you help me?' But no, not you, John! It's not your turn yet! They may find you dead in that booth, but it's not your *turn*!"

I told the nurse.

She took me right in.

The doctor listens to my chest, then rushes me into the EKG room, and that's when he tells me I'm having something . . . but it's very mild.

He didn't use the word "coronary."

But the next thing I know, he's giving me a shot of morphine.


*ANN* I was hanging drapes down in Janice's room when the phone rang. Janice answered it.

"It's some doctor, Mommy. I can't pronounce the name."

I said to myself, Dammit! He left the office and didn't keep the appointment.

I took the phone, and it was Dr. Sofier. "Mrs. Hurley? Don't get upset. I don't want to alarm you."

"Why? What's the matter? What do you mean, don't get upset?"

I can't remember the terms he used, but it was something to do with the heart, and they just took him in an ambulance to Dover General Hospital, and they were calling in a cardiologist who would meet me at the hospital.

And I know I started to go to pieces. Janice came running over and started to cry with me.

My car was in the garage at the time, being fixed. So I sent Janice up through the woods—I couldn't get a dial tone; the line was dead—to my sister Barbara's house. Meanwhile, I got dressed, got out of my house clothes. Barbara came over immediately. She asked me exactly what the doctor said was wrong.

"I forget the term, but he didn't say it was a heart attack."

"Then don't get so upset. It's probably only a warning of some kind, and they got it in time."

She called my other sister, Norene, who lives up here also. By this time, the phone was working again. Norene said she'd meet us.

We took the babies to our neighbor Jane McCormick's house, and Janice went with them.

All the way to the hospital a chill was on me. I silently prayed to God to spare John. To please let him live and not to take him from us now. Over and over I kept saying this to myself.

When we got there the specialist hadn't gotten there yet. I went in to John's room. The nurses were putting all this oxygen stuff on him. I was so scared at the sight of this, I didn't know what to think.

"Don't worry, Mrs. Hurley. There's no need to be frightened.

We're just gonna hook him up till the doctor gets here. This is normal procedure to make it easier for your husband to breathe."

I looked down at John. He managed to smile up at me. I said to him, "Now what in the hell did you go and do to yourself, Hurley?" And he says, "I dunno. But I need a cigarette."

Barbara started to go downstairs to get some coffee for us, and just as she started to leave, the cardiologist got there, Dr. Kroner.

"Would you please all leave the room so that I can examine Mr. Hurley?"

He stayed in with him for quite a while. I was petrified. My mouth got bone dry. It seemed like endless time was passing.

And then he came out and walks over to the three of us. "Which one is John's wife?"

We were standing near the nurses' station. Norene and Barbara were staying back so as not to intrude, and I said, "How bad is it, doctor?" He looks at me and says, "I think you should get his parents up here, just as soon as possible. John tells me his parents are still living. Is that right?"

"Yes."

"We have a priest here at the hospital. Or you can have your own come over."

I couldn't believe what I was hearing. "Why?"

"He's had a massive coronary, Mrs. Hurley."

"Oh my God!"

"I don't think he's going to make it through the night."

"My God!"

"I'm sorry."

I became hysterical. Completely out of control. Started screaming. "Oh my God, not John! We have young children! We have two young babies! They're only infants! He can't be dying! Not my John! Please God, no! Please!"

Dr. Kroner got very abrupt with me. "Take it easy, Mrs. Hurley! Mrs. Hurley! Please! Take it easy! He was shaking my arms. "Mrs. Hurley! John doesn't know it's this bad. He doesn't know he's dying. He'll *hear* you! Now please, stop this and get hold of yourself! There are other patients on this floor! Now stop it!"

I was sobbing uncontrollably. I couldn't help myself. Dr. Kroner grabbed ahold of me and nearly shouted at me. "Goddamn it! Goddamn it, Mrs. Hurley, it's not *you* who's going to die! Now straighten yourself out! Pull yourself together! I don't really give a damn at this point how *you* feel right now! It's *him* we're concerned with. And I haven't told him yet that he's dying."

I still couldn't believe what he was telling me. All I could say was, "He's only thirty-five years old! My God, he's just a young man! He's thirty-five years old! He's never been sick a day in his life."

Dr. Kroner held me firmly, to make me understand. "Mrs. Hurley, problems with the heart have absolutely nothing to do with age."

At this point, my sister Norene, who's a lot more forward than I am, steps between us. I tell her, "He's gonna die."

She looks at me very skeptically. "What do you *mean he's gonna die?*" She turns to Dr. Kroner.

He tells her, "It's a massive coronary. I don't expect he'll live the night."

So she asks him, "What are you doing for him? Aren't you going to put him into Intensive Care?" Which I never would have thought of.

And he says, "We can't. We have no room. There are no beds available."

And she says, "What the hell do you mean, a *thirty-five year old man,* with two young children at home, two *babies,* and you're not going to put him into ICU where there must be people in there who are eighty and ninety years old—that are just *wait-*

*ing* to die?" She got very abusive with him. "I'm not being mercenary, or cruel, but there *have* to be people in there who are so far gone that they can be moved out to save a younger man's life! You oughta be able to take care of him, for God's sake!"

So he says, "Well, you could get a private nurse."

"Would he get the same care?"

And he says, "We wouldn't be able to evaluate just exactly what's going on with him because there wouldn't be any monitoring equipment on him."

"There has to be some way of getting him in there! He's only thirty-five years old. You can't just let him die like this!"

"Age doesn't make a difference when you have a heart attack."

And Norene says, "That's not what I'm saying. What I'm asking is what kind of care will he get if he stays in that room and doesn't go into Intensive Care?"

"Well, we can bring in a private nurse. They're really quite good."

And she says, "How will you know what's going on, what's really going on with him?"

And he said, "There's no way to tell unless we can have him monitored. And that would have to be in the coronary care unit."

"Then goddamn it, and for God's sake, Dr. Kroner, give John a fighting chance!"

"We can't just push somebody else out, like that! Hospitals are not run like that. And I'm sure you wouldn't want them to be."

"Then why don't you at least check? Maybe somebody is ready to be moved tomorrow."

Her voice was getting louder and louder. Dr. Kroner looked at her, then at me, and said, "I'll let you know."

Within half an hour they were moving John's bed into the coronary care section, and they were hooking him up to the monitors. Dr. Kroner tells us, "There was an elderly man that they could take out for a couple of days, to put John in."

I could see why Norene had pushed so hard, because they would have had no way of seeing what was going on inside his heart if he had stayed in that other room.

The priest was waiting for him. He gave John the last rites.

I felt like I wasn't really there, but watching myself in some kind of crazy, nightmare insane dream! It was John, lying there, dying!

As the priest left he touched my arm, to console me.

Norene tells me to call John's parents. I had to get their number from information. John and Esther. His father answers the phone.

"Is Mom there? It's me, Dad. Ann."

"Yes." He sensed a strain in my voice. "Is there anything wrong, Ann?"

"No, I just want to talk to her." I was trying to keep the whole conversation happy sounding, with small talk, so I don't make him anxious. He had a heart ailment himself, and I figure Esther can break it to him easy, and I say, "Mom, you have to come up."

And she says, "What happened? Did anything happen to the children?"

And I said, "It's not the children, Mom. It's John. I don't know how to say this to you, Mom, but . . . it's real bad. He's had a real bad heart attack, Mom. And the doctor tells me he's . . . he's not gonna live past *tonight*! He's *dying*, Mom! Please come up as soon as you can!"

They took the bus and subway and got there late that night.

We all decided to hold off calling John's sister for a while because she lived in Florida and we knew she would want to fly up right away, the minute she heard the news. We didn't want her to make that kind of a trip unless it was absolutely necessary.

Then these friends of ours, Jim and Jean Clark, came up. I was glad to see them. They waited with us.

I spent most of that night walking in and out of John's room, looking at him. He just seemed to be peacefully sleeping. About two in the morning I started thinking of the children, and missing them, and wishing I could see them. I went into John's room with my sister Barbara, and I asked the nurse how he was doing.

"He's resting comfortably."

I told her I was thinking of leaving the hospital.

"How far do you live from the hospital?"

"Twenty minutes to a half hour. I want to see my little children."

"Don't go, Mrs. Hurley. I wouldn't leave if I were you."

That's when I broke down again. "He's really gonna die! He's not gonna come out of it! My God, he's dying! He's really gonna die! I have two babies! Two young babies!" And I know I just kept repeating, "He's gonna die! He's gonna die! Why would God send me the babies . . . after all these years . . . he finally has a son . . . and now He's taking my *husband* from me!"

Barbara was shocked to hear me say this. "Ann! Don't fly in God's face! And don't curse Him! Just follow His wisdom. The Lord works in mysterious ways!"

I didn't know what I was gonna do. I just couldn't face the fact that he was gonna die—and I was gonna be left with three children, all by myself.

John had never been sick before. There was no warning, really. You're never really prepared for something like this. He had had those chest pains, but we had passed it off as nothing. We had pediatricians but we didn't really have a family doctor because neither one of us had ever been sick.

We spent the night.

*The second day.* John was still out of it; he didn't know anybody was there. People were coming and going, all my immediate family, Barbara and Norene, their husbands, my brothers Jimmy and Joey and their wives, my sister Mary, and my parents, and our friends the Clarks.

I didn't leave the hospital.

We called John's sister in Florida. She was there within eight hours.

When she got to the hospital she went over right away and spoke to the doctor. She's a registered nurse. They started using medical terms which I didn't understand. Then she came back to me and said, "Ann, he's a very competent doctor. He knows exactly what he's talking about. And . . . he has no doubts about John's prognosis."

I cried some more. We both cried.

Later I was talking to Dr. Kroner, and my mother-in-law came over and asked, "What is his condition, Dr. Kroner? How is my son?"

"I'm sorry, ma'am, but he isn't doing any better. There's no change whatsoever . . . we still don't expect John to live. I'm sorry. Although he's lived through this one night, it doesn't mean he's going to pull through it. So please don't get any false hopes up."

When he started walking away, my mother-in-law says to me, "Ann dear, don't you think you should have another doctor look at him?"

"Gee, I don't know. He's a cardiologist. A heart specialist. And he seems to know what he's talking about. Joan thinks so too."

"Well, I don't like him. He's got long hair."

"What?"

"I don't think he knows what he's doing. He's much too young."

And she kept this up for the next twenty minutes, until I got to the point where I'm thinking, Well, maybe he isn't too good.

So she and I and my father-in-law went over and spoke to him. And I said, "Are there any complications?"

And he said, "No."

And I said, "Dr. Kroner, my mother-in-law thinks that we should call another doctor in. To get a second opinion." Which, the way we said it, probably was a slap in the face to him.

"Why would you want to call in another doctor? There are no complications. John has suffered a massive coronary. There are no difficulties in diagnosing his problem. It's all too obvious. The man is dying. If he pulls through it, it would only be as the result of a miracle. But he's dying. It's only a matter of time. I have no doubts as to what his condition is. There is no chance of using any heroic measures to try and save him. Believe me, Mrs. Hurley, if I had the slightest of doubts, I would have called in another doctor immediately."

Esther spoke up. "Well, when *my* husband had a heart attack, we had *two* doctors."

"What kind of doctors?"

"My general practitioner, and then he called in a cardiologist."

"Well, that's exactly what has happened here. John went to a GP, and he called *me* in. Look, you can have whoever you want to have. But I happen to be one of the best in the area. You can go up to the director of the hospital, and he'll tell you the same thing." Then he walked away, and left us standing there with egg on our faces.

We let it ride. I stayed at the hospital, and everybody took turns keeping me company. I was never alone at all. My sisters were bringing down changes of clothes and I spent the night again. We slept on little couches for an hour or so at a time. We waited.

*The third day.* Barbara brought Janice down to the hospital. I had told my sister to keep Janice home from school because everybody on the lake knew John was dying, and I didn't want her to hear anything that would frighten her.

I took her aside and explained to her that there was a possibility that her father was going to die. She started to cry.

"What's the matter with him, Mommy?"

"He's had a heart attack—and the doctor doesn't know if he's going to get better or not."

"No?"

"Would you like to see Daddy? He's sleeping. But if you want to see him for a minute, we can tiptoe in."

"Yes. I wanna see Daddy."

Just as she entered the room, there was an extremely nasty nurse there who ordered her out. It's true that ordinarily she wasn't supposed to be in there, but the doctor had given his OK. Janice had just gotten to the door and looked in on John, when the nurse screamed, "Get her out! She's too young to be in here!"

"But the doctor said it would be OK."

"I don't care what the doctor said. I run this floor, not the doctor!"

John was so heavily sedated that he didn't hear any of this. Janice got so upset when she saw all these wires and the intravenous on him, plus the nurse screaming at her, that she ran out, crying. After that I thought it best that she never go back to see him like that.

*The fourth day* I spent it in the waiting room and walking in and out looking at him. The doctor kept telling me, "There's no change, Mrs. Hurley. He's still dying. I'm sorry." I kept telling him, "He's young. He's never been sick before." And he tells me, "Mrs. Hurley, the heart is a very funny thing. If it wants to stop, it stops. All the indications are that he should have died that first night. He never should have lived through that first night."

I was resigned to losing him. But I never *accepted* it.

When he would take a turn for the worse, you could tell. I'd hear Dr. Kroner being paged, and he'd run in to him. John was the only patient he had in coronary care at the time. When he came out of the room, I'd be standing there, petrified.

"No. No. No. Everything's still the same. But we must be realistic. He will be going into heart failure. We must be realistic, Mrs. Hurley."

Or I'd be sitting there with him, and a monitor would sound off, and all of a sudden the nurses would be rushing around, and they'd tell me I had to go out of the room. And I'd go, hysterically crying. And they'd bring him around again. Miraculously.

I always had some hope. And I know I was more afraid for myself than I was for John, to be perfectly honest. I kept saying to myself, What am I going to do? I have three children. Where am I going to go? What's going to happen to them? And to me? Why did God do this to me? He gave me three children, gave John a son, and now He's taking John away from me. Why?

Then, as time went on, I thought, Maybe I'm not seeing the truth at all. Maybe I'm missing the point of it all. Maybe God gave me the children to *replace* John!

I spent all week at that hospital, never leaving John's side.

I slept in the waiting room.

*The fifth day* John came out of Intensive Care. But he wasn't out of danger.

They put him in a room with another man.

For the first time that week, Dr. Kroner was *guardedly* optimistic. "He's still very much in danger. But he is doing a little bit better. But—please, Mrs. Hurley, you must not forget that he's a very sick man. John could still die at any time. Please don't forget that."

I stayed at the hospital all day but didn't sleep there any more.

# 2

## Home

*ANN*  John came home five weeks later. June '71.

That's when the doctor told him he'd have to make a choice —upstairs or the bedroom downstairs. But no stair-climbing—at all—for at least six to eight weeks.

John took the downstairs. He felt it was better because he could walk out in the back yard from the door in our bedroom. He stayed downstairs full time during his recuperation. And it was a bad scene.

He was like a caged animal. He paced and paced and paced and paced—alone in his room—until he got himself to the point where you could just turn the knob on the door and he'd be screaming at you to leave him alone. Screaming. Like a lunatic. I had to keep the door locked so the children couldn't go near him.

He didn't read or anything. Just paced. Every once in a while he'd walk outside for a while onto the lawn and stare into the trees. Then he'd come back in again and pace some more. And he was smoking. Which we didn't know about.

I tried to keep a normal house. But it wasn't. I tried to take care of the kids and keep them away from him, but no matter what they or I did, it was no good. It was wrong. If I stayed with the kids too long, he'd scream. If I stayed with him too long and the kids started to cry, he'd scream. Little John was only ten weeks old at this point and was a very cranky baby. And that didn't sit well with John.

He wanted all my attention. And he couldn't have it. I really had to handle him with kid gloves.

The doctor had him very heavily tranquilized. But it didn't seem to be taking hold. I told the doctor about it. He wouldn't increase the dosage.

We had to see Dr. Kroner once a week, for a checkup. The ambulance would come up to the front door, and the attendants would carry John to the ambulance on a stretcher, and drive him to Roxbury. I'd follow in my car, wait for him, then we'd come back home again. I asked the doctor if this routine was going to last forever.

"I don't think it will, Mrs. Hurley. John is definitely getting stronger. But you'll have to have patience. Just be patient."

So I held my tongue. I never exploded at John, or lost my patience with him, even though I was tempted a hundred times over. I was afraid, petrified really, that he'd have another heart attack.

He became very unfair. He made me feel guilty—very guilty —that it was *my* fault he'd had this heart attack. Me and the children. He said I aggravated him. Me—and the kids, with their screaming and yelling all the time. Said it straight out. "If we didn't have the kids at this time of life, I wouldn't have had my heart attack!"

I was so upset that I phoned Dr. Kroner. I told him that John was blaming me and the children, his young babies, for his problems. "Could it have been that? Could we have been the cause?"

"Absolutely not, Ann."

I think his personality, plus the drive at work, was responsible for his heart trouble. In fact, I'm sure of it. Only a few weeks earlier I can remember telling John to his *face* that unless he calmed down he was gonna wind up at Greystone—which is a nut house—or he was gonna *drop dead of a heart attack*! Because of his nerves!

Before the babies came, John never had to do anything in the house. Never take responsibility. Only his job. That was the only responsibility John accepted. As far as raising the children was concerned, if you'd say, "John, do something," he'd say, "Give 'em a rap! I don't believe in sitting down and talking to kids. Give 'em a rap!"

He very seldom hits the kids. Very rare.

Now, when I went into the hospital to have little John, big John suddenly had a lot of responsibility for taking care of the house. His sister, Joan, came up from Florida, but she's single. She couldn't care less about certain things. If she don't make the bed today, she don't make it. But that doesn't go with John. Everything has to be done to perfection. So he started complaining. He'd get to the hospital, to visit me, and I'd be in a bad mood because he was late, and I'd say, "Dammit John, you only have an hour. Why can't you get here a little earlier?" And he'd scream, "I'm expected to do everything! I'm working all day, I'm running to the hospital at night, I have to go home and cook! My sister isn't doing anything! What the hell do you want from me?"

This kept up for the whole week. Until I said, "Goddamn it, John! Don't bother coming back if you're going to sit here and just complain for the whole goddamn hour!"

Then he'd apologize. "No. I guess it's just me. I'm tired."

But when I took little John home from the hospital, everything just stopped. He didn't bother helping out any more except for doing some grocery shopping, because I couldn't get out with the two babies. One night—I don't know what he brought home, but it was something either weird or stupid. Or both. And I said, "Why in God's name did you buy *that*?" I think it was a giant frozen turkey.

Well, he took it and threw it across the room so it bounced off the wall! Then he screamed, "Do your own fucking shopping from here on in!" Just screamed unmercifully. Then he took the rest of the bag of groceries, and threw them after the turkey!

That's when I told him. "You're a fucking *MADMAN*! You're gonna wind up in Greystone, or you're gonna have a fucking heart attack! I mean it! You're a *MADMAN*! And all because you have to take a little responsibility in this goddamn house! You son-of-a-bitch!"

"I have my responsibility! My job! I bring in the money in this house! And don't you ever forget it! Goddamn it!"

He took his work seriously. It came first. As far as I was concerned, it always came first. I think he was under great pressure at work. All the time. And he never had the opportunity at work to throw something across the room. So that anger came home with him. You could tell when he walked in the door what he was like, if he had had a bad day, because he'd be miserable. If he had a good day, everything was fine at night.

He never talked about work. Very very seldom. Or about the pressure. If I heard anything, it would be through talking to somebody on the phone that worked in Sea-Land. If I would say, "Gee, I heard this one got fired," or just say any gossip that the women knew about because their husbands told them, he'd have a fit. He'd say, "Those women should keep their fucking mouths shut! It's none of their goddamn business what goes on!"

Sea-Land was his private life. No one was to interfere with it. That's how John felt. He'd always treated me that way. As far as his work went, I would say he was reaching a peak of pressure and anger, mostly from work, just before and after the baby was born.

I wasn't so terrific to live with, either. I was miserable. Every little thing would set me off. And he wasn't the type of man that would take the two babies and say, "Why don't you go out for a few hours?" So I was stuck in this house all the time. And I'd say this to him, and he'd say, "They're *your* kids. Don't tell *me* about it." That was his answer to me.

So when he had his heart attack, I was *really* stuck. I wouldn't leave him. The doctor said it was wrong. That I *should* leave—get out—for a few hours. Not twenty-four hours. But a few hours. Just to get away. "He's got to realize that he's not the only one in the world, and he's not the only one in your life. You have a life to lead also."

But I couldn't. I just couldn't do it. As much as I used to get mad at him, I felt sorry for him too.

At the end of the second week—against the doctor's orders—John tried to climb the stairs. Before the embargo was over. He wanted in the worst way to come upstairs.

And he couldn't make it to the first stairwell. I had to help him back down.

He didn't say a word. Didn't say he was tired or anything. Just went into the bedroom, slammed the door, and locked it. He really locked it.

After that it was constantly locked, so the children couldn't get in to disturb him.

If he had company, he'd sit there in bed and have a few drinks. I'd run up and down stairs twenty thousand times, getting things. And as soon as the company left, everybody was put out of the room, and the door was locked again. His room became off limits. His whole attitude would change again.

I don't think he could cope with having two young children around, which is a very hard thing under the best of circumstances. Two babies can be a pain in the ass. Even if you're healthy.

He wanted those kids. At least, I keep telling myself he did. And he keeps telling me he did. But sometimes I wonder if he really did. I've asked him this, directly. He's never admitted that he didn't want them.

I've said it to him. "Just because you didn't want them, or it was a mistake after you had them, you found out after you had them that you really didn't want them, that you don't love them —it's not *their* fault you had the heart attack! The doctor told me that. So don't you lay it on *them.* They're gonna wind up with a complex for the rest of their lives if they pick up on that idea!"

Six weeks passed. We were into July of '71. And John was allowed to climb the stairs *once* a day. So if he came up in the morning, he would have to stay up until he went to bed at night. This went on for another month. We were still stuck in the house.

He wasn't supposed to drive the car. But he disregarded that instruction completely and never let me drive. I've been driving ten years and never had an accident, never got a ticket. But no one drives the car if John's in it.

I would never let him take the children by himself. I told him so. "If you're going to kill yourself driving when you're not supposed to, it will only be yourself. Not my children!"

He couldn't accept the fact of his condition. That this was happening to him. One day, in a particular rage, he said, "Goddamn it to hell! I'm going to blow my fucking head off! You people are going to drive me fucking crazy!"

He was more angry at himself, and so he was taking it out on everybody around him. He was angry at himself for being sick

—and he couldn't wait to get better so he could get back to work.

He got stronger. The doctor said it was amazing. But he made it clear that John must now begin to take things very easy. In fact, Dr. Kroner recommended he quit his job. John blew his stack. "What the hell do you mean, Kroner? No way! I worked one hell of a long time to get where I am today on that job, and I'm not giving it up just because some goddamn doctor tells me to! You oughta have your *head* examined!" He said this right to Dr. Kroner's face.

"John, I'm only trying to be constructive. Either you want to live. Or you don't. It's as simple as that. What's the difference if you're a shoe salesman or an executive, as long as you're *alive*? I'm not saying you should never work again. I'm just saying you should be working closer to home, in a less demanding occupation."

"There's a goddamn big difference, Doctor. I *worked* to get where I am, and I'm staying where I am. And I intend to go further. I didn't work all these years to put in what I put in and then wind up with *nothing*!"

**JOHN** So then Dr. Kroner suggested that we move closer to work. He felt that the commuting was bad for me.

"What if I were to take the *bus* and not drive to work?"

"No, John. It wouldn't make any difference. You're sitting immobile, and that's very bad for you. It's no good for *anyone* to be commuting on a daily basis for a distance of a hundred and forty miles a day. That in itself puts a hell of a lot of stress on you."

But to me it was relaxing. The driving. Except when you had a real snowy or icy night, and you're all over the road, and these nuts come flying by, or some nutty woman in front of you slams on the brakes! Other than that, it was relaxing. Never bothered me. I sort of preplanned my work before I got to the office, by thinking to myself while I was driving.

He wanted me to quit the job, come up here and even sell shoes or something. He says to me, "What's the difference?"

So I said, "Oh no, it doesn't work that way, Doc. I have no life insurance except what I have through the company. And now I have a heart attack. I can't buy any life insurance. And let's face it, I'm used to living at a certain standard. There's no way I can quit my job now and still support my family, the house, and everything else in the style to which we've become accustomed. No possible way. Financially, I'm not in a position to quit work."

So he says, "You've got to measure your finances against your life."

And I said, "Well, Doc, I'll take my chances. I've got to keep working at Sea-Land because that's where all my eggs are."

He said, "If you'd come to me a year before, I would have told you you were a sitting duck for a heart attack. The driving, the stress, the strain, the exertion. You were just a sitting duck."

"It's very easy for you to sit back and make hindsight pronouncements, Doc. But let me ask *you* something. If it was you and not me, would *you* retire?"

"John, if I could, I would *tomorrow.*"

# 3

## *No Hope*

*ANN* We started looking for a house down closer to work. In August. And we couldn't find any. I saw a couple I liked, but John would never agree, never give his approval. I just think he didn't want to give this house up. So Dr. Kroner said that if he got air conditioning in his car, and centrally air-conditioned the whole house, he could go back to work. That meant selling the Mercedes. A blow to his ego. He had bought the car without air conditioning, because he liked the way it looked, and the dealership told him they couldn't recommend installing it afterward, for mechanical reasons. Of course they'd be happy to sell him a new car. So I talked him into a station wagon. It's more of a family car, and more economical.

He went back to work. It was September. Three days a week, half days. He'd go in after the traffic, and come home by three in the afternoon. Sea-Land accepted this with no problems. And his salary remained the same. They were very good about this.

Then, after a couple of months, he increased his schedule to four days, then to five days.

By January, he was back on full time. And making his business trips as well. He'd have small relapses and some discomfort. But they wouldn't hospitalize him. He just shrugged it all off.

A year passed. Then he started having chest pains. Dr. Kroner said these were angina pains, and put him on nitroglycerin. That's when they put him into Beth Israel Hospital for tests. To see if a coronary bypass could be performed on him.

Several leading men examined him. Dr. Parsonette, Dr. Zucca, and Dr. Rothchild. He spent a weekend in the hospital. Put him in on a Friday, and he came home Monday. God forbid he should miss a day of work. He felt that, even if they wanted to, he wasn't going to ever let them operate, because he'd read everything he could get his hands on about coronary bypass operations and heart disease, and he felt that the operation wasn't generally very successful. But I talked him into at least going for the tests.

As we were leaving, the doctors forbid John to drive, because of the drugs and dyes he still had in his system. They were firm. As we got to the car, I said, "I'll drive, John. You take it easy." It was like waving a red flag.

"Oh stop it, willya? I'm all right!" He could have killed us, the way he was weaving in and out of traffic. "I'm all right! It's these other lunatics that don't know how to drive!"

Two weeks later, John was home from work and went out for a walk with the baby, for his exercise. I called Dr. Kroner to find out if he had gotten the results back from the tests.

"Yes, Ann. I just got them back today. Is John there?"

"No. He's not here. He's out taking his exercise."

"Ann . . . this is going to be pretty hard . . ."

"What?"

"Ann . . . you're going to have to mentally prepare yourself . . . for what I have to tell you."

I got frightened. "What do you mean, mentally prepare myself?"

"Nothing can be done for John."

"You mean the arteries are that bad?"

"I mean there is just no hope. They've given him *maybe* six months. Ann, it could possibly be *two years* if he takes it very easy."

I said nothing. I would have just babbled if I opened my mouth at that point. I was trying to understand what he was telling me. The finality of it. I just couldn't understand it. It wasn't real to me.

"When can you both come down to the office? I'll explain everything to you in as much detail as I can, to give you both the clearest possible picture."

And then I said, "No . . . no . . . you cannot tell him."

"He's got a right to know, Ann. He's my patient, and I think he should be told."

"Dr. Kroner, I'm his wife . . . and I think I know John best . . . and I've got to have the last say on it . . . and no way in hell are you gonna tell him this. Really. I'm going to insist on it."

"Well . . . you know John best. But think about it, Ann. I won't say anything until you let me know."

And I said, "It's definite. I've made up my mind. I'm *not* going to tell him. I don't think he could handle it."

I hung up the phone, and something in me just gave way. I started crying hysterically. Sobbing uncontrollably. I felt worse than I ever had before. Because I had felt that he was really doing well, and I had grown hopeful that everything was gonna be OK. And now that hope was gone.

I called my sister Barbara.

"I just got the results of the tests he took at Beth Israel. They say he's gonna die." I was crying now, full force. "The baby won't ever know him. His son will never know him! Little John will never know his father!" I don't know why, but that part of it sticks in my mind.

"He will, Ann. There's enough of us around, there's a lot of photographs, the family is close, and they'll always be wanting to tell him what his father was like." Then she said, "I'll be right down. I want to be with you."

"You can't. John is going to be home in a few minutes. I've got to stay calm and get myself together. Because he can't know."

And she said, "I won't say anything. I'll just tell Ronnie when he comes in."

John came back from his walk, and then it was a big pretense from there on in. Pretending everything was OK.

I never did tell him.

He continued working.

It was impossible for me. Every time he went out I never knew if he would be coming back again. But I felt I owed it to him. I really don't think that John would have been able to handle it. I think he would have died before he should have. And I don't think I'd want to know if I was gonna die.

There were times when I lay awake at night, crying, after he fell asleep. Just looking at him. And to make sure he was still breathing.

We were still having sex. I'd be frightened. I was afraid it was gonna overwork him.

The doctor constantly asked about our sex life, but said, "Don't worry and don't get a hangup about it. There's nothing wrong with it. It won't kill him."

But I was afraid. I was petrified he'd overwork himself and die.

But John didn't think about it at all. It didn't faze him in the least. Never thought about the strain. He would've said, "It's a terrific way to go, anyway!"

It was terrifying for me.

I think those were the worst moments of my life.

# 4

## The Two of Us

*ANN* We met in a bar. In 1956. The Norwegian Dance Hall. In Brooklyn. Park Slope. I was sitting with my girl friends, Bonnie, Alice, Ann, and Pat. We were sitting there, drinking beer, and he comes walking in and says hello to my girl friend Bonnie.

"Hiya, Bonnie."

And I said, "Who's he? He's cute."

And she says, "Oh, that's just some kid I went to school with."

We were around twenty. And he offered to buy us a drink. The four of us. So we all ordered rye and soda. And he shit. He really did. He gave us a dirty look and said, "I thought you were drinking beer!"

And I said, "Not when someone else is buying!"

That was the first time we met. We started dating, and a year later we were married. In St. Michael's Church. The same church I was baptized in, and received the Holy Sacraments.

I grew up in a family of nine. Five girls and two boys. We lived in Brooklyn, in Bay Ridge, and I attended parochial school. Then I went to Bay Ridge High School.

When we were first married we had fun. We had a good time. We didn't have children for the first two years. We went out a lot and went away for weekends.

I was working for American Machine and Foundry, doing general clerical work. John had just gotten out of the Navy. He went to work for a steamship company.

*JOHN* I got out of the Navy February of 1956. We were married August of '57.

I had all intentions of becoming a lawyer. I was going to night school. CCNY. The Bernard Baruch School of Business. Under the GI Bill. Taking a full twelve credits.

My business drive at that point was nothing. When Janice was born, I was forced to change jobs because we needed more money. From that point on is when I developed the attitude that I really had to put out.

Before Janice came along, Ann worked and I worked. So we shared everything. On weekends we cleaned the apartment together. I felt that as long as she was working, fifty percent of my responsibility was inside the house too, and if that meant cleaning up as well, then I accepted it. But when Janice came along, I felt my responsibility was to provide the *means*—and Ann's was to provide the *motherhood.*

Janice was born with a dislocated hip. One leg would have been shorter than the other because her thigh socket was not going into the hip socket properly. I hadn't been in my job at American Hemisphere long enough to be covered under their medical and hospitalization insurance, for Janice. Anyway, we were fortunate in that the doctor caught it right away. But the bills started mounting. I had to drop out of school and take a second job, to pay for her medical expenses.

Janice wore braces until she was seventeen months old, and then she walked perfectly. But until then, we had to take her for weekly treatments—to an orthopedic specialist. And at that age she kept growing out of the braces, which were very costly.

I was majoring in law, with all intentions of going to law school. And I had a very good opportunity. I belonged to the Maritime Lawyers' Association. You could have someone sponsor you if you worked in that field, which I did, because I was a claims agent, and all of your claims are handled either between insurance companies, or with lawyers. So I was working intimately with lawyers and the law, even though I wasn't a lawyer yet myself.

*ANN* He was a *swinger* too, in those days. Chasing girls. I caught him a couple of times. Not in bed. But I caught him sort of making *plans*. There was a woman I worked with who was old enough at the time almost to be his mother. A good fifteen years older than me. But she was a swinger. She made a play for John. This was five months after we were married. At a Christmas party for the office I worked in. The party was at the Bay Ridge Manor. They were making a date to meet the following day, and I had come up in back of him, and he didn't know I was there. And as soon as I heard what was going down, I went over and said, "Sweetie, I'm gonna drag your ass from one end of the street to the other! No one steps on *my* toes! If you want to get out, John, then get the hell out all the way! And don't come back! And God knows, you can do better than this *dinosaur*!"

I didn't play around, so I didn't see any reason why he should!

But he didn't feel that way. John feels that women are second-class citizens. He really and truly does. That we're second-rate. He's his own man. He has his ways. And that's that.

There were other women.

One time, when I was pregnant with Janice, we were at a friend's house, on Shore Road in Brooklyn. This was just after a wedding ceremony. I had been upstairs at the time, in the ladies room, and John was downstairs at the reception, setting something up. I started walking downstairs, and a friend of his who knew what was going on all of a sudden comes over to me and is stalling me with small talk, to keep me from coming downstairs. He was obviously trying to stop me from finding something out—but I happened to get a side glance in a wall mirror and saw John bullshitting some chippy. So I pushed his friend aside.

"Get the hell outta the way, goddamn it!"

I stormed over to the two of them. John was shocked to see me, and when he saw the look in my eyes, he swallowed hard. I didn't care who was there. I was furious. I didn't care where we were. I cursed John out in front of everybody. "I'm not a fucking whore like that bitch is! I'm not spending another minute here with you, you dirty rotten bastard!"

And I stormed out of the house. He comes running out after me and says, "Ann! I swear it! She was just offering to mend my socks!"

I couldn't believe my ears. I saw red.

"Fuck *you,* mend your socks. You *bastard*!"


**JOHN** We moved from Brooklyn to New Jersey, because Janice was growing up and we needed a house. I felt that we should get away from the city and move to a suburban area. And things were very rough at that time. Could just about afford the house. We used to go out once a year. On Easter Sunday. That was the only time we could afford to go out.

My background is all steamship and transportation. Before I

joined Sea-Land, I was a claims agent for American Hemisphere. Strictly marine cargo claims. It was great experience. You got to know what the world is really all about.

They were having a lot of problems with theft at each one of their ports. They had their own agents at these ports, but thefts were becoming so commonplace that they couldn't be sure if the *agents* were in on the stealing or not. So they sent me out to investigate. This was '62. I went from New York to New Orleans, British Honduras, Guatemala, El Salvador, Nicaragua, Costa Rica. Virtually every port and country in Central America. All of them.

First, I would be incognito, watching them discharge the ship, and checking the goods off the ship. I'd usually disguise myself slightly, dress up like an old man, or a tourist, so as not to attract attention to myself. Then, when I saw what was going on, and who was doing it, I'd move in. In the majority of cases, the customs officials themselves were stealing the cargo. These tin-badge crumbs were robbing us blind. They had confederates who were diverting the goods under their jackets, into pushcarts, into new crates with different forwarding addresses on them, into waiting taxicabs, Volkswagens, bicycles, and even army trucks!

Then I went to Sea-Land Service. This was still '62. As a manager. I was twenty-seven, and a workhorse. The average employee age at my level was thirty-five.

My job encompassed responsibility for all of the Caribbean Islands, including Puerto Rico, as far as cargo losses were concerned. Let's say your company shipped something, and an item winds up damaged or missing. You'd file a claim, and my responsibility would be to process and investigate, to determine whether or not you're entitled to payment. And you had to put in the hours. But there was an esprit de corps in those days. It was a very closely knit company. Everyone shared that feeling. Someone was always willing to help you with your problems, and you them. When you went with Sea-Land, it was more like joining a family.

In 1964 Sea-Land moved us to Puerto Rico. We faced some tough challenges down there. The primary problem stemmed from the fact that when Sea-Land first started its original operation in Puerto Rico, the intention and agreement with the government was that we would agree to have local PRs as managers.

But after letting them run the operation for three years, everything got so fouled up you couldn't believe it. It still boggles the mind. First of all, we had PRs handling the cargo who didn't know how to properly handle or deliver it. And it was like this all the way through the entire operation. Incompetence.

So the company put together a team of managers—nine of us gringos—to go down there and straighten the whole bloody mess out (and simultaneously try and educate a Puerto Rican to be your ultimate replacement). We worked our asses off. Seven days a week. Fourteen, fifteen, sixteen hours a day. For the first whole year. Straight. Never had holiday one.

I was threatened many a time by the Puerto Ricans. If they didn't like what you ordered, or if they felt they were being pushed too hard by the gringo Americanos, they'd grab two-by-fours, and start swinging! There was one of our guys, Hank. They creamed him. Put a two-by-four *between his ears.* Made apple sauce out of him. Down in old San Juan. On the old Waterman Piers. Another of our guys was shot up and is still a cripple. He'll never be normal again. They hung a sign on him afterwards which said "YANKEE GO HOME!"

You're dealing with an element. I'm not talking about the PRs in general. Only the longshoremen with no education whatsoever. They're animals.

I got threatened by the *customers,* too. For example, we'd ship a load of tomatoes down to the island. And the shipper finds out all of a sudden that the market for his tomatoes, the bottom has dropped out. So what he does is, he claims they're all *damaged*. He comes to the depot, has one of his boys pull out the plug or tear the wires out of the refrigeration unit, and he'll say right to your face, "Hey! Looka here, Señor Inspector. No function!" This bastard is looking you right in the eye. "This no good, Señor. No function. *Tomato malo!*"

Until you tell him, "Look, pal, we delivered that trailer to you and it was working just fine. Now the wires are all cut. That's *your* responsibility, buddy, not ours!"

So this guy is sitting there with maybe a twelve-thousand-dollar loss, which is not Sea-Land's responsibility but his own problem with the market drop, and he'll straight out tell you you're gonna be found in the street with your *balls* cut off.

After that first year a bunch of us used to pal around together when we had a day off or something, and they used to call us the "Wrecking Crew." One of the guys down there was from Cuba, Ricky DeJesus, and he lived above this bar in this big apartment complex, and the bar was called the La Rue. It was the favorite hangout when we finished working. We'd stop by and have a drink before we went home. One night, we had an out-of-town visitor. His name was Thompson. And he wanted to see the Puerto Rican operation. So we showed it to him! We took him out that night to see the sights, and all ended up in this La Rue. And they had a band playing. Guys with the mariachis and the pleated shirts. And the Desi Arnaz faces. Well, when the band took time out, we went up and *nationalized* their instruments! And of course there are like eight or ten of us, so the musicians didn't feel like making a formal protest. So we're playing away! I grabbed the drums, Jim Clark the sax, another guy the piano. And we were wailing! Thompson had that scratch thing you play. And we sounded like *SHIT*! Unbelievable!

The next day we come into work, and we're all hung over, heads hammering. And Ricky DeJesus, he wasn't with us that night, but he lived upstairs, and we got to talking over the coffee pot, and he says, "You know, I gotta move outta this goddamn apartment I got!"

"Why, Ricky? What's the matter with it?"

"Last night, in that little bar they got downstairs, the La Rue? You shoulda heard the *racket* that was coming out of this place! Madre Mia! Such *poo-poo!*"


*ANN* In a way, we had it made in Puerto Rico. We paid two hundred and fifty dollars a month for a private house. You could get a live-in maid for next to nothing. A gardener was five dollars a month. We had four bedrooms downstairs, two bathrooms, a living room, dining room, and kitchen. Upstairs was another bedroom and separate bathroom, and in the back was a separate maid's quarters.

Like any normal wife, I was just fed up with the idea that John was either at work, or was out taking a client out for entertainment on the town. I never saw him. He wouldn't get home sometimes until three or four in the morning.

Once I found a letter in John's pocket. From a girl. Saying that she enjoyed being with him—and that she wouldn't bother asking him any more questions about his married life, pumping him any longer. She was saying that she would take him on his own terms. It was almost divorce time.

I had been going through his pockets, looking for tickets to a dance we were supposed to go to. I was supposed to take the suit to the cleaners, and I wanted to take the tickets out of his pockets. Subconsciously he must have wanted me to find it. The letter was addressed to him c/o Sea-Land. And underlined, in red letters, were the words "personal correspondence." The minute I saw it, I knew it was a girl's handwriting. When I asked him about it, he swore (and still swears to this day) that a friend of his wrote it, just for a joke. To see if I would find it—and see how much trouble it would start between us. Of course that's just a crock of bullshit. That's almost like the "mending socks" routine! Mending socks! A classic!

I knew that letter was the real thing because John had said earlier in the month, during an argument we were having, something like, "I don't know if I want to be married or not." I asked him what was going on, and he said, "I just can't make up my mind whether I want to be single or not." So I put two and two together.

I remembered that for a couple of days earlier that month I had been unable to find out where he was. He had gone up to the States, supposedly to buy a new car. I hadn't heard from him in two days, and nobody in the States had heard from him. I knew he had quite a bit of cash on him and I was worried that something might have happened to him. That he might have got mugged or something. So I called his office, to find out where he was. And everybody put flyers out on him. And he had a *fit* when he got home to find out I was checking up on him. But I wasn't. I hadn't any doubts about him, and no reason to check up on him —I thought. I was just afraid that he might've gotten mugged with this money on him.

So several weeks later, when I found this letter, I put two and two together—that he had been with this broad. And I flew home. To my parents.

It wasn't a legal separation. But I felt I should come home for a while, to sort out my feelings. Apparently I was more mentally disturbed than I thought I was, because I went to my priest, Father Coogan, at St. Michael's, and I spoke with him about the problem. He asked me if I had any proof that John had gone to bed with anybody.

"Well, he's come home with lipstick a couple of times on his collar, but he tells me it's from innocently dancing."

Father Coogan told me that this was not proof positive. And if I loved John, I should forgive it, forget it, and put it out of my mind. But I'm not that type of a person. I'll go to my grave with it.

But after a while, I just couldn't stand being away from John. He would call me and ask when I was coming back. Then he'd put it this way, "If you don't come back soon, Ann, you don't have to bother coming back." Charming. But I didn't budge. At first. "Then stay in Brooklyn until *I* decide what's gonna happen!"

So finally, I went to my doctor about it, because the doctor knew both of us for years, and I explained the whole situation to him about the letter, and about John's decision that I should stay in Brooklyn until *he* decided what we're supposed to do. So he says to me, "Ann, what the hell are you supposed to do? Sit in a rocking chair until *John* decides what *you're* gonna do?"

I said, "I really don't know."

"Well, I think you'd better lay your cards on the table—and he better make his move. Don't sit home waiting for him to make up his mind. It's *your* decision to make. So make it."

And when John came up on a business trip, he apologized to me and said he was sorry for the whole thing. And I guess I must have believed him. That innocent smile of his has probably gotten him out of more scrapes! I went home with him, convinced everything was OK.

Looking back, I'm not sure that I believed him, or just convinced myself that he was telling the truth. But I'm sure he really *was* sorry that he had caused this problem. At least sorry that he had gotten caught.

I can forgive. But I never forget.

*JOHN*  In 1966 we were transferred back up here to the States again. That's when we moved up here to Forest Lakes. Nine years ago, Halloween.

Come '69, Sea-Land was having one hell of a lot of losses with the military. This was during the height of the Vietnam War. There was a bunch of thieves, between the GI's and the Vietnamese and the crooks who ran the commissaries and PX's. Things were disappearing like crazy. The trouble was mainly in Vietnam, but in order to investigate the problem, we had to go just about around the world. We left New York and went first to San Francisco, to see the military out there, because they alone had filed something like four million dollars' worth of losses in one clip. So we investigated their claims and said, "There's something definitely wrong here. In fact, this is horseshit!"

I suspected what was going on. Let's say a trucker came to California and delivered 100,000 cases of beer. You could only fit maybe 40,000 pounds of those cases in one of our trailers. So it would be broken down into 20 to 30 trailer loads of beer. So we'd ship them over to Vietnam—and what would happen is they would check out from each trailer how many cases they supposedly received. Well, if one trailer was manifested that it had 1000 cases in it, and it only outturned with 900, the military would claim 100 cases *short*. But if the next trailer parked alongside of him was manifested with a thousand cases, and it outturned with *1100* cases, they wouldn't credit the 100 cases that were *over. Someone was making off with the hundred cases!* The guy in charge of the PX *was making out like a bandit!* We finally and conclusively proved it.

Our investigation was a great success. We photocopied the Army's records and then proceeded to put the onus on *them.* Over and over, they had claimed that they just never received *x* number of shipments. But the disposition was that we had them by the short hairs. They were forced to drop a hell of a lot of claims, and face up to the pilferage that had been going on. The company saved *millions* of dollars on that trip.

On the way home, we stopped off in Honolulu, and I reported to my boss by telephone. I had cabled a full report ahead. And that's when he asked me if I'd like to become Director of Special Commodities. I was floored. This was a major step up for me. I immediately told him yes.

When I got home, I told Ann about it. She was pregnant with Joan at the time. And she flipped out. She was tremendously excited and happy about it. We went out to dinner that night at the best restaurant in town. Naturally we had lobsters and champagne. And then, so help me, we, or I should say I, topped off the evening by singing, out loud, with my champagne glass hoisted high—and everyone staring at me as if I was crazy, and Ann trying to bury her face in her napkin—I sang "America the Beautiful"! Came right *out* with it! " *'Oh beautiful, for spacious skys, for amber waves of grain. For purple mountain majesties—'* " Oh, let me tell you, it was lovely!

I received a substantial raise in salary, plus bonuses, and incentives tied directly into revenue generation. Beautiful money.

My responsibility could be stated simply. I had to coordinate all of the trailer loads, to make sure that all the equipment Sea-Land owned was placed at strategic locations, at peak seasons. Six thousand five hundred refrigerated trailers, worldwide, generating upwards of one hundred million dollars in gross revenues, annually, to the company. It was one giant chessboard.

We called our headquarters building in Port Elizabeth, New Jersey, "Disneyland East." It was spotless. Immaculate. You could eat off the floors. Beautiful, modern brand-new building. My private office had a screen enabling me to keep tabs on all of the trailers, telling me where they were allocated, and for what purpose. Each day I'd update it. My window faced out onto

Newark Airport and the New Jersey Turnpike. And I could watch the jets taking off and landing all the time. My desk had a telephone with a lot of multiple lines and an intercom for my secretary.

Each office had its rubber plant, which was watered daily by the maintenance people. The size of the plant was your status symbol, signifying where you stood on the totem pole. Mine was pretty fair-sized.

The business is extremely competitive. On produce, your customers are working on pennies sometimes. And meats—they could be working on a quarter of a cent per pound. So it's gotta *MOVE*! If the cargo isn't delivered in a certain time, the market can drop, and the customer can lose his drawers. And you've got fierce competition between different transportation companies. It's a constant battle to be first with the most. Guys are calling you up and saying, "How come you give this guy fifty-five trailers today, and you only give me forty-five? What kind of bullshit is this?" So it's a bit of a pressure job.

When I arrived at the office in the morning, I was immediately presented with maybe fifteen problems, because the world is still spinning, twenty-four hours a day. Fifteen hairy problems that *had* to be solved. That's exactly what it boiled down to. And you'd have five different salesmen waiting to see you, all ready to jump on your ass to find out why you couldn't take care of their customers. Eight-thirty in the morning. "John, we've got eighty-eight loads booked for that ship—and I've been told you're only gonna have seventy pieces of equipment! How are you gonna get me eighty-eight pieces to cover my eighty-eight customers?" So the day didn't build. It just started with a *BOOM*!

You see, the salesmen would call on their prospects and say, "Do you have any freight you're gonna move this week?" And the prospect might say, "Yes. I need five trailers." So the salesmen would say, "OK, we'll get you five trailers. No problem!" So he goes to his branch manager (let's say in the Jacksonville, Florida, Division), and says "XYZ Company needs five trailers next week." Sounds simple enough, right? *Sure* it's simple!

But maybe one of his trailers breaks down, and winds up in the garage. Now he can only supply *four* trailers. In the meantime, the customer has set *all* of his internal business based upon those five trailers he's been promised. He's signed contracts to sell five trailer loads. He's ordered enough lettuce, say, to fill up five trailers. But now he's only got four. What the hell's he gonna do with an extra load of lettuce sitting around, that he's already contracted to sell but he can't move—because we can only supply him with four?

Well, the first thing he does is pick up the phone and get ahold of the goddamn salesman. The salesman then gets ahold of his manager—who gets ahold of his counterpart in corporate headquarters, and says, "Hey! I told you I could make ten reams of dough on this deal, but I don't have the equipment! You didn't give this guy sufficient equipment!" So then his boss would come screaming to me.

"Hurley! Goddamn it! What the hell is going on? How come we can't give this guy—who owns forty-two farms and is one of our best customers—one lousy extra piece of equipment?" So you'd say, "Hey! Hold on! Who the hell could tell that truck was gonna break down? There it is, sitting in the garage." Then you'd jump all over the maintenance manager's ass, trying to get that unit repaired in time to be of service to the client. And the maintenance manager might say, "Hey! This isn't my fault! The factory can't supply the replacement parts right away. They're on back-order."

It's a snowballing effect. I guess I was the end of the line. The buck definitely stopped at my desk.

Sometimes the static went all the way up to the president of the company. He'd call me and say, "Hey, John. How come you can't give these people the equipment they need? What happened?" I'd usually have my feedback by then so I was ready for that phone call to come down. I would break my *chops* to find a replacement for that equipment, but if I couldn't do it, no one could do it. The president's tone was always polite and understanding. But he would just want to make sure that you checked every possibility, thoroughly, and that you knew who was on *his* ass.

At about eleven in the morning, many's the time I'd get the feeling, What am I *doing* here? What the hell am I *doing* here? This is *fucking crazy*! So we used to go out and have two or three martinis at a cocktail lounge nearby, with our lunch, to sort of relax a little.

Because it never let up. Never stopped. Even after I left the office at six-thirty to drive the seventy miles home, and get home by eight, that phone would still be ringing before I had a chance to sit down for dinner. Because you're working around the world, with all the different time zones. So they'd call me at all hours. Europe and the Far East would often wake me at midnight. And there'd be some guy who had a problem. "We need sixty-three trailers additional to cover a contingency." And what are you going to do? Alaska calling. Thailand. Seattle. Calls from all over. London. Haiti. And everybody needing everything *yesterday*.

But I never thought of getting out of the business. Never. Because the higher you go, the less problems you have. You have *bigger* problems. But there are *pauses* in between. A laborer is taking fifty shovelfuls an hour out of a ditch. His foreman might take a shovelful every hour, just to show how it's done.

Now that I think about it, though, the weeks before my heart attack were a ballbreaking time for us. It was that period of time when all of the annual division budgets and projections had to be finalized. The completion date was March 31st. I had my heart attack three weeks later.

# 5

## *The Secret*

*ANN*  I never told him that he was dying. John thought everything was all right. Dr. Kroner never specifically lied to him. He just told John that the damage to his arteries couldn't be repaired with a coronary bypass. John accepted it. But the doctor told me I should begin mentally preparing myself to be a widow. This was February '73.

And right after this John thought this was a perfect time to get away from everything for a while and take a cruise to the Caribbean islands! I was terrified. I didn't want to go. He didn't know how sick he was. He became insistent. He wanted to go in the worst way. I just wanted to keep everything together, right here. And I didn't want to take him away from the children. I thought a trip like that would be too strenuous, too much on him. I gave him no indication that I knew anything was wrong. I just told him, "You know I hate water. You know I'm petrified I'll get seasick." That carried no weight.

Jim Clark called me from work, to scold me for my attitude.

"What the hell's the matter with you, Ann, you don't want to go on a cruise with John? It'll do him a world of good after how sick he's been."

And I just said, "Oh, Jim, I'm so afraid of boats bobbing around, and sinking in all that water. If I'm gonna go, I'd rather go fast."

All his friends thought I was terrible that I wouldn't consent to go.

We flew to San Juan, then got on the cruise ship for the islands. And right after we set sail, he got chest pains. He couldn't breathe properly. Couldn't catch his breath. We were sleeping, and suddenly it hit. The first thing he wanted to do was get out of our cabin, go up to the deck, and get some air. He just about made it upstairs. He sank into a deck chair and just sat there, gasping for breath, trying to catch his breath and breathe deeply.

"John, you've got to call the ship's doctor!"

"Forget that, Ann. I don't need him."

"But John, you're in trouble. For God's sake, let me call him!"

"Absolutely not! And I don't want to hear any more about it!"

"But why? Tell me why!"

"Ann. Did you get a good look at him? The guy's Italian. He sounds like Chico Marx, for crissakes!"

"You're crazy! You know that? You're sitting here, you can't even catch your breath, you have a known heart condition, and you're refusing to see the ship's doctor because he's *Italian*? I can't believe you're in your right mind!"

"I'll be all right. I just have to take it easy, that's all. This is only a minor problem. I'll be all right."

"John . . . I'm worried. I don't like the way this looks. I'm worried about you. I'm scared. Please see the doctor."

"Look, Ann. First of all, the guy can't even speak *English*! I'm not gonna let that son-of-a-bitch tamper with me! You don't know *what* the hell he's liable to do! And if he was any good, then what's he doing on a cruise ship? Why doesn't he have a practice of his own. Hah? Answer me that!"

"John—"

"If I was seasick, or I had a headache, I might go to a doctor like that. Or a hangnail. Or if I needed an Ace bandage! And besides, what can he do for me? I'm already taking nitroglycerin to ward off the angina. So what else is he gonna do for me?"

I thought they were gonna take him off that boat in a wooden box. I never told our friends Jackie and Mike Ladner, who were on this cruise with us, just how bad John really was. I really believed this was it. He was gonna die. I was convinced it was definite—I would be bringing him home dead.

We walked the decks all night long. He couldn't stand to be inside the cabin. We had to be outside. Every single night. Struggling to breathe. Sometimes during the day it would subside, and John would try and enjoy himself. He was determined to see that cruise to the end. There was nothing for him to take for the breathing. The nitroglycerin didn't help. It was heart failure. I wanted to call in a helicopter, so that we could be flown back to the States for treatment. He absolutely refused.

The ship went from San Juan to St. Thomas, Martinique, then back to San Juan. It was a beautiful cruise. The food was out of this world, the service just first class all the way. And it was just a catastrophe. John couldn't eat, and he couldn't sleep. One hour a night, tops. As soon as everybody went to bed it would hit.

The Ladners could see that John was having a problem, but since John obviously didn't want to talk about it, they didn't pry. Mike Ladner was definitely worried. "Ann, I think John ought to see the ship's doctor. He looks . . . his face is very pale. Don't you think? I don't like the way he looks, Ann."

John felt like he was suffocating. He couldn't get enough air. He was very white and pasty. Every time the ship docked at an island, he would get out for maybe half an hour, trying to walk and sightsee. But he couldn't make it. He could barely hold a camera steady enough to take a picture. I'd see his hands begin to shake, and look at him. He'd look at me, and we'd excuse ourselves. The Ladners were great about it. We'd go back to the ship and wait for them to return.

He'd be very quiet about it until everybody went to bed. Then we would go out onto the deck. He had to fight to breathe. He would stand at the railing, and just *pull* the air into him. Every once in a while he'd clutch at his chest. I could see he was in severe pain. But he was a determined man. You could not argue with him. It was *his* life, and he was gonna live it *his* way. And that was that.

When the ship docked back in San Juan, I begged him again to see a doctor.

"Ann, *for crissakes,* just leave it alone, will you? I'll handle it! I'm not going to any Puerto Rican doctors. I don't *trust* Puerto Rican doctors. If I didn't trust an Italian, you think I'm gonna go see a PR?"

Etta and Lincoln Blakely, friends of ours from Sea-Land, met us at the dock, and that night we went with the Ladners to a party at their home. They were marvelous hosts and served a wonderful meal. Everyone was laughing and having a great time. Except John. He looked like he was at a funeral. He had to force himself to smile.

When we flew back from San Juan for home, he was in real trouble. But he wouldn't even let me tell the airline that he was having a problem. It was as if he were denying its very existence, by refusing to acknowledge it.

We got home on a Sunday.

His mother had been babysitting at our place. When John went out to visit a friend, we sat down to talk. She asked me how we had enjoyed the trip. John was still resisting calling the doctor, and I thought maybe his mother could help. I told her he had had a very bad time on the ship. And that I was worried about him.

"Oh, Ann. Don't worry. It's probably because he was drinking too much. Or smoking too much."

"No, Mom. It's something much worse than that."

"You're probably getting worried over nothing."

"It's not nothing, Mom. It's very serious."

She looked at me strangely. I think she thought I was exaggerating my fears.

"Mom, the doctors up at Beth Israel gave John a series of tests, to find out how bad his condition is. And to see if they could operate to maybe correct it. And they can't. They told me that the damage is so bad that there's nothing anyone in the world can do for him. This was three different doctors up there, Mom. And they all said the same thing. He's dying. He's got maybe six months more to live. Two years at the maximum, if he retires. Which he refuses to do. But he's dying."

She looked at me like I was out of my mind. She flat out didn't believe it. "It's not true. There's some mistake."

"No. We saw some of the best doctors on the east coast to try and repair him, but they can't do anything for him. They took tests to see inside his heart and arteries."

"There's some mistake." Then she started to cry.

John and I went to Dr. Kroner Monday morning. He checked John over thoroughly. Then he gave him some water pills. And said he had to retire.

"Immediately. No ifs, ands, or buts. You have to retire immediately."

"What about for a year or so more?"

"John, there's no two ways about it. I'm sorry. I'm telling you as your doctor that you've got to retire. You cannot work any more. It's just as simple—and as serious—as that. You're having heart failure. Your heart is not pumping enough blood through your body. It's a combination of things. There's not enough oxygen getting through, and you're building up fluids all the time."

"What about six more months?"

"John, if you want to believe that, I can't stop you. But your heart is giving out on you. I'm telling you for your own good. No more work. *You've got to retire.*"

John cried all that night. He just went into the bedroom, locked the door, and buried his head in the pillows, sobbing. I've never heard him like that before or since.

He went in to Sea-Land the next morning and went straight in to see Jim Clark. "Jim, I have to give you two weeks' notice. The doctor says I have to retire."

Jim couldn't believe it. John had been looking and feeling so well.

"The doctor says my heart is even worse. Maybe I can come back in a year. I'd like to hope so. But right now, I'm afraid that I just have to call it quits. And retire."

The doctor never told John that he could ever return to work, but John kept right on believing it.

Jim told him, "Don't wait two weeks, John. You'd better go *now*. If it's that bad, I don't want you traveling back and forth to work. Your life is more important than any goddamn job."

He and Jim went to the personnel office to find out what he was entitled to, and what he had and what he lost if he went out on disability. And after he found out that he still had all his medical and life insurance, he called me. He sounded emotional.

"Ann, I'm coming home. I've checked everything out, and we'll still be provided for. I'll be on half salary for the rest of my life."

Then he cleared out his desk and left.

# 6

## Out

*ANN*  As soon as he hung up, I called Jean Clark. I cried to her. And I told her the whole story about the tests and all. And she cried with me.

"Ann, why didn't you tell us before this? Why did you keep it a secret? Why did you keep it from us?"

"Because I never told John what the doctors had said. I never wanted him to know. And I didn't want anybody to ever *tell* him." I knew that the more people you tell, the more it gets around. "John should have retired a long time ago, Jean. He's dying."

She told me she would explain everything to Jim, and that they would be in touch with us.

John drove home. And no sooner did he walk in the door, he poured himself a beer and got on the phone. He called my two sisters and my brother who live in the area and asked them if they wanted to go over to the Adam Todd, which is a very nice restaurant over here, for dinner. There were a few grumbles.

"Jeez, John. Everybody's working. It's the middle of the week." Those kind of grumbles.

"Listen, pal. It's my *retirement dinner*. I *retired from work today*. And if you can't go tonight, forget it."

And everybody went. Bobbie and Ronnie, Jimmy and his wife, Miriam. And Norene and Bernt. And John and I. And he wouldn't let anybody else pick up the tab. We had champagne of course, and everybody was told to order whatever they wanted to eat and drink.

He told the waitresses and the maître d' he was retiring, and acted very happy about it. They came with a huge cake with frosting on it which read "congratulations on your retirement." When the waitress brought it, she looked around at all of the faces. "Who here is retiring?"

And John pipes up, "I am! I made my first million! And I promised my wife I'd retire when that splendid occasion rolled around!"

She stood there, looking at him beaming. Then she looked at me and said, "Really?"

And I said, "Yeah. Really."

This is how he is. You have to keep laughing. With a flourish. John had always said he'd retire at thirty, a millionaire. That's what he used to tell everybody. So my sister Norene calls him on it. "You bastard! You *did* retire! OK, so it was a little past thirty. So where you hidin' the million, John?"

It was a wonderful party. John made sure that the strain didn't show. There were a lot of laughs and kidding around. John toasted himself. "To a wonderful person, who got out when the gettin' was good."

Everybody went along with it.

The next day was the first day, as they say, of the rest of his life. He had a box of his personal belongings that he had taken from work when he emptied out his desk. His friends told him that he should come back for his stuff later on. But he took it all that last day. And he has never set foot back at that office yet. His friends have asked him and asked him and tried to make arrangements for lunch, but he's never gone back. He just can't face them. And he's never opened that box of stuff yet. I've asked him a hundred times to sort it out so we can get rid of any junk. He just says, "Leave it alone, Ann."

This was March 1973, and it was a nice time of year.

John took up fishing. And for the first couple of months, he adapted very nicely. He would relax and fish, and he had friends in the area who are firemen and would be off two or three days in a row, and they would all get together and play cards. Then he knew some men who were older than he is, some of them are on disability, and he'd hold conversations with them over at the tavern.

But once in a while he'd get frustrated that no one was really on the same wavelength with him. That they really didn't have that much in common as far as business and the stock market were concerned. That's when he became interested in local township affairs and joined the planning board. He became vice-chairman.

Until now, Sea-Land was his whole life. He had never talked about anything else.

The planning board reviewed site plans, subdivisions, and master plans for the township, to make sure the builders complied with all the local ordinances and standards. He was appointed by the mayor.

But every so often he would have a blue day.

# 7

## Fear, Money, and Anger

*JOHN* When I first had to go on disability and leave Sea-Land permanently, that's what hurt the most. You've left the job and there's no possibility of going back to it. It's final. The doctor didn't hold out any false hope. He just said, "John, you've got to face this. You're finished with work. You cannot work any more. Period."

I'm sure that people who are forced to retire at sixty-five, the same feeling goes through them. I'm one of the people who'd work until I was eighty if they'd let me. But something else hurt, too. There's a hitch in my disability income which I didn't know about until some time later.

The company's disability payments are tied in to my Social Security payments, to equal exactly 50% of my base salary at the time of my retirement, minus incentives and bonuses. But when Social Security came out with a recent 8% increase, as a cost-of-living escalation, I got an 8% *decrease* from the insurance company!

It seems that there was a loophole written somewhere in the policy with the company. I got a letter from the insurance company stating that this is specifically mentioned (in the fine print, of course) in the contract with Sea-Land. They were thinking ahead when they wrote that contract and were already prepared for cost-of-living increases before they were even passed by Congress!

Therefore, it's conceivable that, if the cost of living keeps going up (as it inevitably will), in a few years, the insurance company will not be contributing a goddamn red cent to my income! It will be strictly Social Security that'll be supporting me.

I suddenly realized that I could *never* get ahead. I'd always be behind, because the cost of living always goes up. My blood boiled. I realized that we would just about make ends meet. Maybe go out to dinner once a month. Cover interest and amortization on the house. Pay for food and utilities. And that was it. *We were screwed.*

I immediately wrote to my congresswoman, Helen Meyner, in the hope that the government might be able to help us. She took it up with the Commissioner of Social Security, James B. Cardwell, who wrote me a letter explaining what the reasons are for it (it's cheaper for the employer) and that they're trying to do something about it and hopefully they will, but at present there are only three states where legislation specifically prohibits the insurance companies from doing this. Massachusetts, New York, and Illinois.

Beautiful!

But basically, my argument is with the insurance companies. I think they're making a windfall on these things. I think it's a crime. I really do. I think it's a goddamn shame. I wasn't aware of this at all, and I'm sure a lot of people haven't read the fine print in their insurance contracts, either. So what are you supposed to do?

And it took two years after I went out on disability to become eligible for Medicare! Can you believe that? At my age there's a two-year waiting period. There are one hell of a lot of people who retire at sixty-five in perfectly good health. But if someone else goes out on a medical disability at a younger age, the reason they're going out is because they're *sick*! So who would need medical assistance and attention more?

And we were not eligible for two years. I don't understand the rationale at all. If it were up to the government, you'd *die*.

This time of my life required an enormous adjustment. It was exactly what Dr. Kroner said. "John, you've been an active person all your life. You've never been forced to be home twenty-four hours a day. When you were working, you probably saw more of your coworkers than you did of your own wife and family. So the one thing that you and Ann will both have to adjust to is finding something diversionary to take you away from each other during the day. You cannot spend twenty-four hours together. It's impossible. You're going to get on each other's nerves, and it could lead to a divorce." He was absolutely right.

So the first thing I'd do when I got up in the morning was get the hell out of the house! I'd just tell Ann, "Pretend I'm at work. Pretend I'm not even *here.*" Fortunately I enjoy fishing, and we live right up here by the lake, so I'd get up in the morning, go over and sit on the boardwalk with a six-pack of beer and a sandwich, and I'd fish from nine in the morning to three in the afternoon. Then I'd come home and I'd have to rest.

Being home like this was an unusual circumstance for a man to be in. Sitting out there, alone, for hours and hours, nobody to talk to. I'd see the planes flying by overhead, and I'd automatically associate it with work. I'd say to myself, "I wish the hell I was on one of those planes. Going *someplace*!" I thought about that a lot. All the trips I used to take all over the world for the company.

There were a lot of things running through my mind. Memories. And the feeling of shame, or guilt, of being in this condition. And not being where all the other men are. Men are not supposed to be home between nine and six every day. We have a society rule, and people look at you in a strange way if you're around the house at eleven in the morning.

I thought it was very funny for a while. Everybody else was going to work, and I was staying home. I made a big joke to myself about it. But it stopped being funny after a while. I still relate myself to work. Even to this day. I still keep in contact with what goes on at Sea-Land, what changes they're making, and who's going where, and how the organizational structure is changing. And I wish that I was down there being a part of it.

I missed work tremendously. The day I left for good, there were a lot of people I never even said good-bye to. I was too emotional, you might say, to really go in there and talk to them. Because it came as such a shock. I couldn't understand why it happened to *me*. As I walked out to the parking lot, I saw some guy walking down the street, and he's 400 pounds. Obese. And I said to myself, Jeez, look at this guy! He's obese! The fat's just running all over him! He's almost got *tits* and everything else! By all the odds, he's the guy that should have had a heart attack! What the hell did I have a heart attack for? Why *me?* Why *me,* and not some lousy stinking hippy goddamn draft dodger who won't even serve in his country's service? Why are these little fags walking the streets, and not me?

You wonder why something like that happens to you. You become obsessed with finding an *answer.* A reason. Something you can *live* with, to make you understand. But there is no reason, really. And when it does happen, it's *there.* There's nothing you can do about it. There's no way of turning it around. And it eventually dawns on you.

For a long time I kept insisting to Ann that it was a dream. A nightmare. A terrible nightmare. Everything happens so fast that you just don't believe that it's happened at all. You say to yourself, Jeez, this can't be true! This can't be *real.* This can't be happening to me!

But it was all too true. And real. It was all over for me. I was out. Out of Sea-Land. Out of my job. Finished. Forced to clear out my desk. Forced to relinquish my command.

I guess I was pretty bitter about it for a while.

# 8

## The Childhood Years

*JOHN*   I was born in Brooklyn. November 27, 1935.

My parents are John and Esther Hurley. I have one sister, Joan, who is two years older than I am. She's a nurse. We've always been very close.

My mother is Norwegian. Both her father and mother are Norwegian. Name of Pederson. They're Protestant.

My father's side is French, Irish, and Scotch. Stanch Catholics on my father's side. Church every Sunday, novenas, missions, large families. My father's brother Eddie, up in Maine, he's got eight children. I was raised as a Catholic.

My father was born in Maine, graduated high school, and left at an early age to get a job in New Jersey. His philosophy was that when you left high school, you were sort of on your own, and he brought us up that way. I don't feel that way toward my own children. I'm more protective. My sister has always felt that we were sort of pushed . . . not shown the affection . . . and were sort of made to feel that our mother and father were waiting for us to get out and be out on our own.

My father was a machinist. Tool and die maker. For as long as I can remember, he worked for Permudil, a company that made water softeners and purifiers. Tool and die makers are renowned for not making a good dollar for the experience and the technical background they have. Even today. So money was tight. It was a problem, no doubt.

My mother was working. In fact, as long as I really can recall, my mother always had a job. She worked for a long time in a doll factory. Then she went to work for Lord & Taylor, as an elevator operator.

When I was a baby, my sister, Joan, was my protector. She always took care of me wherever we went. We always got along very well, and we always depended on each other.

We lived on Fifty-seventh Street, between Eighth and Ninth Avenues, in the Park Slope section of Brooklyn. It was a six-story building. Our apartment consisted of two bedrooms, a living room, a large hallway, and the kitchen. My mother and father had one bedroom, and my sister and I shared the other. Until we were eighteen.

I was very skinny. They were forever giving me vitamin pills. And calling me Sonny. My aunts still call me Sonny.

I had a number of jobs as a kid. I delivered the *Brooklyn Eagle,* shined shoes, and delivered groceries on Saturdays, worked in John Wanamaker's department store after school. Delivering the *Eagle* was a pain in the ass. Because I didn't have a bicycle. I *walked* my route—which was a considerable distance. I had to walk from my house to Fiftieth Street and Sixth Avenue, where they had the little office where you'd pick up your papers. And walk from there to Sixtieth Street. I had the route from Fourth Avenue and Sixtieth Street, to Sixtieth Street and Eighth Avenue! On *both* sides of the street! A considerable walk with the *Eagle* bag. Especially if you remember the *Eagle,* how thick it was.

I had two best friends, Matt Kune and Davey Oborg. Davey lived next door to me. Matt lived a block way. In fact, both of them were at my wedding party. Another fellow was Eric Chell. Another Norwegian. These guys were from a Lutheran background.

As a child I actually was friendly with two groups. One was a group of Norwegians. Very religious. I was the only Irishman. Matt, Davey, and Eric belonged to that group. And the other group was "Moosh" Balduccio and his tougher group, consisting of Italians, Irish, and Portuguese. Moosh was Italian. Vinnie Calandra was my best friend out of this group. This was a rougher group.

The first group, the Norwegians, we'd play basketball down by the church. They all belonged to the church basketball team. With Moosh and Vinnie, it was another type of a thing. Altogether. We used to get into one hell of a lot of trouble. Forever getting into street fights. Fifty-seventh Street against Fifty-eighth Street. The Apaches vs. the Eagles, and you'd better stay the hell off our turf. That type of a thing.

We used to hang out on the corner, shoot the breeze, play cards, or play ringolevio, stickball, marbles, mumbley-peg. With your pocketknife. You'd have to drop the knife off of your knee, your nose, off the top of your head. Your finger. Sometimes I'd come home with a black eye. Next day I'd come home with both my eyes black. It was a rough type of a neighborhood. I used to get my shellackings.

To make extra money, Vinnie and I used to go to the junkyards. We used to get the pushcarts, leave a dollar deposit—they had a two-wheel pushcart—and we'd go collecting newspapers and old rags.

It used to take the two of us to get that cart off the ground. One guy would get on one side of the handle, and the other would get on the other side, and you'd go through the garbage in all the cans in the neighborhood. All the cans.

You'd have stacks of newspapers and rags, four feet high. Then you'd take everything back to the junkyard, and the junkman would weigh it. They paid by the weight. Rags used to pay the most money. And they paid us *zip* for it. So we'd wet the bottom layer down to add a few pounds.

Must've weighed a coupla hundred pounds by the end of the afternoon.

Afterwards, there was this Jewish bakery, "Osky's." They made the best rye and pumpernickel bread, rolls, and bagels at this Osky's bakery up on Fifty-eighth Street and Fort Hamilton Parkway.

At night, what we used to do is we'd go up and buy a quarter pound of butter, we'd chip in for it, and when the freshly baked bread come out of the ovens, they'd set it on long tin racks to let it cool.

And we'd sneak in, and grab one off the rack, and run like hell!

And then we'd cut the top of the bread off with a pocket knife and stick this quarter pound of butter in the middle of it and just let it melt and sit under a street light and play cards and eat this bread.

Delicious!

We did this more than a few times. In fact, whenever we felt like it. Which was pretty often.

Either Vinnie or me would get the brainstorm. "Let's go up to Osky's. I'm hungry!"

Today, if my son or daughters did the things I did as a kid,

I'd break 'em in two. It's a different world. Today, you're very protective, for some reason. And you never heard of this dope problem. Maybe a few musicians smoked reefers, but it just wasn't popular with the kids. It was more alcohol. Beer or booze.

This Italian kid, Moosh, his father would put up barrels of wine in his basement. After school we'd go down there and we'd drink like fish. It's probably the first drunk I had in my life. Moosh's father was the only one who owned a house. Mr. Balduccio had a very good job, managing a trucking company, and those kids never wanted for anything. They never worked or anything. They're probably a bunch of bums today.

Anyway, we used to go down to his basement all the time, and, like the French, the Italians used to have wine with their meals. We were drinking wine out of cheese glasses, and I had maybe a dozen glasses of this wine and wasn't used to drinking at all. I came home *stoned*. Just *stoned*. Trying to act sober. And I'm eating dinner, and I get sick as a dog. Ran away from the dinner table and threw up *everything*. My old man, he comes into the toilet where I'm retching my guts out, and he lets me have it. WAP! Took one look at me and knew what the hell I'd been up to. WAP! WAP! He always knew. My father was a firm believer in law and order.

We had a girl in the neighborhood, when I was twelve, who was twenty-one. And she was a cousin of Moosh's. She was also a nymph. Name of Angel.

We used to take her down to Moosh's finished basement. He had a younger brother, Jimmy, who I was very friendly with. And there was a guy named Lenny. Wore glasses. And another guy, Wally, who always wore Keds. So we'd take her down to this basement. She was very willing. And we used to sit there and drink wine. And all of a sudden, someone would flick out the lights, and we'd "attack" her. Actually, she'd attack *you*! She was really beautiful. Thin. Brunette, large brown eyes, great boobs. Fantastic legs. Fantastic!

This was my first sexual experience, was with her. These meetings might have anywhere from three to nine guys there at a time. She was a good teacher, was very kind, and made it very easy on you. There was no doubt she was a nymphomaniac.

Actually, this had been going on for quite a while when I hadn't known about it. But one day Jimmy says, "C'mon, Hurley. We're having a party. And Angel's gonna be there." So I say, "Is this the one you guys keep talking about?" He says, "Yeah." So I say, "OK. I'll be there."

The first time I ever went down there, I just sat back in amazement and watched. They'd turn out the lights, and before you know it she'd have all her clothes off, the guys would too, except some socks, and I just sat there. At first I thought maybe they were pulling my leg or something and they wanted me to grab her, and then they'd all sit back and laugh or something. So the first one I sat out, in the bleachers. Thereafter I was a participant.

She finally moved out of the neighborhood, to Staten Island.

I didn't go to parochial school. All public schools. Went to PS 39, then to PS 105, and then I went to Pershing Junior High. I used to play a lot of hookey when I was in junior high. My sister and I would sign our parents' names to the attendance cards that the teachers sent home. Since we got home before our parents did, we could always intercept the notes. We did this for almost six weeks. Finally, the school sent a serious letter home. "Mrs. Hurley: Your son John has been out of school for 45 days. We would like to schedule an appointment for you to come in and discuss this matter." My mother beat the hell out of me. She didn't wait for my father to get home. Then she went up to school and told my teacher that she was working, and that's why we were out and unsupervised.

Then I went to William Grady Technical School. And I got thrown out of it. Expelled. For knocking out a teacher.

I was going to become an electrician when I got out of Pershing. So I went to Grady Annex, just past Coney Island, where they had one floor with machine shops set up, and electrical shops, and I was going for electrician.

Vocational schools were rough in those days. They really consisted of people that couldn't make the grades to go to an academic school. And while I was going there, there were these two Italian guys—one was a little, sawed-off runt named Baboush; and the other guy, his cousin, was a big guy, bigger than I was, with a clump of red, matted hair, name of Big Red. He was probably two years older. He looked like he didn't belong in school. More like he should have been in the Marines. So we were just starting school, and this guy Baboush was a troublemaker.

We used to use these icepicks—like you'd wire a whole complete house on a wall, on a miniature basis, and to start a screw in the wall, you'd use an icepick. So everybody in the class had their own icepicks, to start with. Which was kinda dangerous. So to start the screw, you'd just jam the icepick in the wall and start your screw, and take your wire and wrap it around to outline the whole house. Then you'd hook it up to a battery and bells, so the teacher could check all the circuits out.

I had just finished my assignment and went to the bathroom. And I come back and this little Italian, Baboush, had torn my whole project—wires, battery, bells and all—right off the wall! Just before the teacher was to grade it! I almost died. I worked so hard on it. So I look around, and Baboush has this punky grin on his face like he's daring me to start something, and he's got an icepick in his hand.

"Summata Hurley? Fuck up your house or somethin'?"

Well, I just went over to him and put him up against the wall and began to drastically change the features of his face—and the next thing I know, his cousin Big Red comes over and grabs me and spins me around, and I'm taking these two monkeys on at the same time! The class goes ape!

With this, Mr. Herzberg, our instructor, comes over to try and break it up, and while I'm taking a shot at Baboush, Mr. Herzberg steps right in front of it—and *POW*! I hit Mr. Herzberg *right in the mouth*! Well, his dentures go *flying,* and he goes up, over a table, and down over some chairs, flat on his back—*out cold*!

So all three of us go marching up to the dean's office. And even though they knew those guys were the troublemakers, they threw us all the hell out of school. Gave us our walking papers. That was it. You just don't go knocking out the teacher.

My mother called up Fort Hamilton High School to find out if there was any possibility of my finishing school up there. We went up to see the principal, and they took me on a probationary basis. I was warned: The first time I got into trouble, out I went. So I graduated Fort Hamilton High School, in 1953.

It was a different world. Kids today have it a lot easier than we ever did. They have a lot freer life. And they don't realize it. Every Saturday that came around, you were working. If it wasn't shining shoes, it was working in the grocery, delivering packages, or in Wanamaker's, or delivering telegrams, or the *Brooklyn Eagle.*

You were hustling. It's a fact. You were forced to. You really were. Because that's the only way you had any source of income. If you wanted something, you got it for yourself. I'm not saying this was extreme poverty. It certainly wasn't. Millions of kids were brought up like I was in that era. Your folks gave you *the basics.*

And a lot of hand-me-downs. I can recall going down to some house on Thirty-ninth Street, where the guy we used to get our clothes from lived, a friend of the family. He was a truck driver, and he used to have a lot of additional clothes and produce and appliances from his truck which he used to sell on the side—and also his kids had extra clothes which they had outgrown, and we used to go down there and get *their* hand-me-downs. I can remember it.

It was a big thing if you went out and got brand-new clothes. It really was.

# 9

## Dying

*ANN*  This "retirement" of John's went on for almost two years. We adjusted to the financial cut of 50% salary. We sat down with pencil and paper and figured out that cutting out commuting, clothing, lunches, parties, and a new Mercedes every two to three years made a real difference right there.

It was hard for me to accept the fact that he was home. I was resentful—because if I had someone in for coffee, or for lunch, they wouldn't come over any more after that. Even when *good* friends were here, having coffee and conversation, when John came home from fishing and announced that he was going to take a nap, they would invariably leave within a few minutes. They felt awkward.

I said to John, "I really wish you'd let me know when you're going to be gone! I'd like to have some kind of a life of my own!"

And he'd say, "I'm not stopping you."

But he was. Completely. Without realizing it. Or meaning to.

I was afraid to leave him—even for a few hours—because I never knew when he was gonna go into heart failure.

In July of '74 he started to deteriorate. He was rushed to a nearby hospital. They gave him the last rites.

The police chief up here is Eskil Danielson. And he's usually the first one at the house when John has to take an ambulance to the hospital. When you call the Lakeland Emergency Squad, an alarm is sounded by radio to all of the volunteers, and Chief Danielson must be monitoring the radio, because he's usually the first one at the house. This has happened eight times already. He's actually carried John into the ambulance.

I'd be downstairs with John, and the way the house is laid out, it's almost impossible to get a stretcher up the staircase to the front door, because of the turns. So they generally carry him out into the back yard from the bedroom, and then up the sundeck. Then the chief calls ahead to his patrol cars and has the roads cleared for us so that the ambulance can go right through. He has his siren going in front of the ambulance, clearing the traffic, and they get John right to the hospital.

John sank.

They treated him.

He recovered.

They sent him home.

I'm not being callous about it. It just was the same kind of thing he'd gone through before. Only the dates were different.

In August he got very bad. We were getting ready to go down to the beach. We were having a beach party, and suddenly he started looking kind of pale.

"John, what's the matter?"

"Nothin'."

You could always tell when something was wrong because he got this funny look on his face. Pasty. Very pale. And I said, "You're having a problem, aren't you?"

"Oh. A little bit. It's getting a little heavy in my chest."

"Maybe we should call Dr. Kroner?"

"No. Let's wait a little while."

He went downstairs to lie down, and it was getting worse. Then it would pass. Then it would come back. Then it would pass. Then it came back again. I said, "I'm gonna call Kroner." He said, "No." But I called him anyway.

The first thing he asked me was what his color was like.

I said, "Very bad."

"Then he's not getting enough oxygen. Take his pulse."

I did, and it was way too high.

So he says, "Ann, get the ambulance right away."

I did. Then I called Bobbie, and she and Ronnie came up right away. Ronnie takes me aside and says, "Oh God, Ann, he looks real bad this time."

And I said, "He really does. He looks worse than he did last month."

He was sitting in a living room chair, trying to look as if he were comfortable, and everything was all right. Typical.

The ambulance men rushed in with oxygen, and John *brushes them off*! "Naw. I don't want it. I don't need it."

I was frightened. The last time I had been able to insulate myself a little bit from it. Trying to be strong. But now I was frightened again. Janice went to her room, and I could hear her crying. Joanie got her blanket. And little John was confused. "Not feeling good, Daddy? Not feeling good? Please feel good, Daddy. Please feel good. Want *ice cream*? Wanta *ice cream*?"

I suddenly realized that every time the ambulance pulled up the driveway, the baby had thought it was the Good Humor Ice

Cream truck! John managed to smile at me, he thought the baby was so adorable.

But this one was a bad turn. Heart failure again.

At the hospital, Dr. Kroner took me aside. "Ann, I know you've heard this before. But this time . . . I think we've got to be prepared for the worst. It really doesn't look good."

"Do you think I should call his parents?"

"If they want to see him while he's still alive, they'd better get here pretty quickly."

I called them. But I didn't try to convince them to fly up. By this time they had moved to Florida. I just informed them of John's condition and told them I'd keep them posted. They sent him their love.

John received the last rites. This was the sixth time. After a while I almost lost count. And this time, the priest scared the hell out of him.

John was coming in and out of it, and the priest was in the middle of the ceremony. All of a sudden, the priest remembered that he had forgotten the oil to anoint John with. So he left the room for a minute, to fetch it. And John wakes up to find this misty-looking shrouded figure—in black—coming over to him from out of the shadows, ready to anoint him. Well, John sat straight up in bed! The priest jumped three feet backward, scared *pink* himself! And John is looking all around him to make out where the hell he was. Then he looks at the priest and says: "Don't DO that! You scared the *hell* outta me!"

Miraculously, his condition improved. Eight days later they took him out of ICU and said he was doing well enough to be put in his own room in another wing.

One day passed, and they were going to let him go home. I brought his clothes with me to pick him up. But when I walked into his room he was in severe pain again. He couldn't move, he couldn't breathe, he couldn't sit, he couldn't get out of bed or stand up.

I kept calling the nurse. She said she'd be there in a few minutes. He was getting worse, and I was getting more nervous.

He had so much pain in his chest it was agony for him to take a breath of air. And he was so distressed—he could barely *lie down.* The hospital was extremely good, but the nurses were just so busy and I guess they thought he was a complainer, I don't know, so they had neglected him. He looked terrible. He was white. He was gasping. I said to myself, What the hell's going on here?

I ran to the nurses' station. "Something's wrong! Something's wrong with my husband! He can't breathe! You have to give him something! *Immediately!*"

And the nurse looked at me and said, "I can't do a thing. The doctor isn't on the grounds right now, and I can't get in touch with him to give your husband anything."

I wanted to strangle her.

"You better get something in there to him *now*! There's something drastically wrong!"

And she got very huffy, and says, "You'll just have to wait."

So I went downstairs to the telephone booth in the lobby and I called the doctor's office and spoke to him myself. "I don't know what the hell is going on, but John can't breathe, he's in severe pain, I've told three nurses, and they all tell me either to *wait*—or they're all going off duty!"

Dr. Kroner had by now gotten very personally attached to John. "Don't worry, Ann. I'll take care of it."

And by the time I got back upstairs, the nurses were in his room. They were obviously annoyed with me for having called Kroner. They never said anything, but they were very arrogant toward me. Told me I had to get out for a while—and I told them I wasn't leaving the room.

Dr. Kroner rushed in, took one look at John and said to the nurses, "My God, what happened here? He's going downhill again." They just stared blankly at him.

This shows you that if you don't open your mouth, you can lose the battle right there. John had been in pain for five hours, and the nurses just kept telling him to wait and wait and wait. *He had a clot in his lungs!*

Dr. Kroner put him back in ICU. The priest came in again and gave him the last rites.

I really felt for sure then he was gonna die. I said good-bye to him while he slept.

But two days later he started to pull out of it. It was miraculous.

Dr. Kroner said, "Thank God, Ann, that the clot didn't lodge in his heart. Normally, it might have, and it could have killed him. But it seems to have passed right through—and lodged in his lungs. But we're not out of the woods yet. There may be other clots that we don't know about. He's in a very critical condition."

They kept him very quiet in bed for another ten days. Then they put him in a semiprivate room, and in a few days, he came home.

*JOHN* I found myself thinking about suicide. Not that I would actually do it. But I couldn't help thinking about it. I think someone who does commit suicide is temporarily out of their mind. Anyone that takes his own life has to be in a real demoralized state of mind. If they weren't in that state of mind, it would take a hell of a lot of courage to do it.

There were times . . .

One thing I had always said to Ann was, "Ann, if I ever end up having to spend the rest of my life as an invalid, bedridden,

I would be capable of taking my own life. I might really do it. There would be no doubt in my mind that I *could* do it."

I told Ann I knew exactly how I was gonna do it. I said when I was cleaning my hunting rifle, it would accidentally go off. She made sure the gun was never near me because she didn't know for sure if I really meant it or not.

But I always made sure I knew where she hid it.

We started having some juvenile problems down at the lake. This was August of '74. A bunch of kids from another township started trespassing onto the beach, which is private, and waking me up at night. They started coming over here with these hot rods, drinking, making out, screeching out here, really tearing up. Happened time and again. And I couldn't get any sleep. I tried yelling at them, but it didn't do any good. So I called the cops. But these kids had CB radios in their cars so that when the police dispatcher would be sending cars over, the kids would pick it up and immediately take off. They were never around when the cops came.

I was talking to Chief Danielson one day and telling him about it, and I said, "You know, Chief, I hope you don't think that I'm a crank, or that I'm crying wolf when I call in to complain about these kids coming up here, because every time your policemen come over here no one's ever around." And he explained to me that he knew about the CB radios. Because he knows all the kids in the area, and who the troublemakers are.

"John, do you recognize any of the cars? Do you know whose car it is? Or what make and color it is?"

"No, Chief. It's too dark at night to make them out. But I'll tell ya, the next time they come by, I'll *mark* them for ya!"

"What do you mean you'll mark them for me? How?"

"Oh, I'll think of something."

The next night they were back, hootin' and hollerin' like wild Indians. I couldn't get any sleep. They were really dancing it up with their music blasting.

They started getting to me. I got really angry. Ann was still sleeping. I went to the storage closet, took down my 12-gauge from where Ann was hiding it behind some blankets, loaded both barrels, went out onto the lawn, and fired two warning blasts into the sky!

"Now get the hell outta here, you little bastards—before you really get me angry! *MOVE IT!*"

Those kids scrambled out of there so fast you'd think a herd of elephants was charging them.

*Ann* almost had a heart attack when she heard the shots! She woke up out of a sound sleep and ran to the door to see what was going on, and when she saw me with the shotgun, she ran over to me just as the last of the cars was disappearing down the road.

But they never came back.

Toward the end of '74, I started getting this congestive heart failure type of a thing. And it was really bad. Progressively worse. From August to October I was in and out of the hospital, maybe twice a month.

And then I fell off the boardwalk. While I was fishing. This was the end of October. I cast the line and I just *fell over*—right into the water! It was as cold as a well-digger's ass! The water was twenty feet deep there, and I had all my clothes on. Heavy winter clothes. But there was a tree floating in the water, and I grabbed onto that. I don't know if I passed out, or if I slipped, or what. It was scary.

But the shock of the water revived me, and somehow I managed to haul myself up onto the beach. I lay there, panting, soaked, exhausted. Must have been there for half an hour, shivering in that freezing cold. I kept working my fingers and toes to keep them from icing up. It was so cold I almost couldn't stand it.

*ANN*   I caught sight of him coming up the hill from the beach, with his soaking clothing, and his hair all matted to his head, the water still dripping off him. He looked like something out of Boris Karloff and *Tales from the Crypt*. He was shivering cold. I got him out of his clothes and made him towel down and quickly put pajamas and a bathrobe on. He slumped into a chair in the bedroom. I poured him a drink. He couldn't shake the chills. And he couldn't stand up. I knew it was heart failure again.

I called Dr. Kroner. The ambulance came for him and took him to the hospital. Janice couldn't come with us because she got so hysterical and frightened. So her friends Ellen Berkowitz, Lynn Mazzucca, and Linda Torkelson came over to stay with her. The Traegers and the Woods took care of the little ones.

There was another patient in the room with John. He was at least 350 pounds, about fifty years old, and he had no legs. He was watching us when Kroner came in.

John knew he was dying.

"What's going on with me, Doc? Tell me. Give it to me straight."

"I *would* like to speak with you, John." His manner was very grave. "John, I'm gonna level with you. You're not getting any better. Things are really getting very much worse at this point. And you're going downhill . . . fast."

He paused for a second, as if to measure his words.

"John . . . Ann . . . I've been in consultation with a number of other doctors, cardiologists . . . and because I'm afraid we've exhausted every other possible alternative . . . I really think that we'd better begin to seriously consider *a heart transplant.*"

John just sat there. Didn't say a word. The fat guy across the room is watching and listening to this and doesn't know where to look or what to do with himself. I could tell that because of the way he was fidgeting nervously; he didn't think he should be listening to this, but he couldn't leave the bed or move his curtain with his no legs, so he watched us, very uncomfortably, from across the room.

I started to cry. The tears were building up and rolling down my face. John was totally and completely stunned.

"But I'm only *thirty-eight years old*!

"I know."

"Is it really *that bad*? Don't I have *any other choice*?

"No, John. I'm afraid not. I'm afraid you have no other choice. Except of course, to do nothing."

I was in shock. *A heart transplant!* I couldn't believe Dr. Kroner was really saying it. It's just something that you'd never think of. Maybe you read about it in books and magazines. But for John? *A heart transplant!* I was dumbfounded. It was surely the end of the road.

"I want you both to give it some serious thought. Think about it very carefully."

The tears were just rolling out of me. I couldn't help myself.

John says, "Let me ask you something, Doc."

"Yes."

"If it was *you,* would *you* do it?"

"John, I can answer you two ways."

"What do you mean?"

"If it was my *father,* who is seventy years old, who was in your condition, I would say no. Right now, I'm two or three years older than you are. If *I* was in your condition, and the rest of my health was good, I would say yes. I would try *anything!*"

"Yeah."

"But I have to explain one thing to you. You must understand this. I can *try*—only *try*—to get you into the hospital program where they do this kind of surgery. It doesn't mean they're going to definitely operate on you. We just have to play it by ear and see if they'll even consider looking at you or examining you. They may say no, right from the start. I can only *try* to get them to evaluate you as a candidate for surgery."

*JOHN* I was pretty shook up. Dr. Kroner must have seen it from the look on my face. Because when he left he said, "Is there anything that I can have sent up for you—special?"

I said, "Yeah, Doc. Do me a favor, will you? For once in my life, I'd like to have a *drink* in this hospital. A nice, real, tall, ice-cold *alcoholic beverage!*"

I'd asked him many a time if I could have a drink or some wine with my dinner, and he would never go along with it. But he did that night.

"What do you drink?"

And I said, "Scotch."

So he says, "Well, you can't have soda. But how about Scotch and water?"

"Just gimme the Scotch, Doc."

So he did. I had two drinks that night. And you know something? Thinking about a heart transplant was the same *after* those two drinks as it was before they got to me! I guess this was the first real sign—even though I'd suspected—it was the first time I really *knew* I didn't have much time left on this earth, when he suggested the transplant. From that point on, you sort of weigh things. Carefully. All the alternatives.

Now, I've been just about everyplace. I've seen a lot of things.

I've done just about everything there is to do. There are still a lot of things I *wanted* to do. But if I was a bachelor I probably would have said no to the operation. When your time is up, it's up. That's all. But the biggest thing I had to consider, and the reason I believe that I decided to go through with it, was not for my own life extension. It was more for the benefit of my children. Because at that time, my son was three, and my daughter, the little one, was four. I thought I owed it to them more than anything else. That's the way I felt.

Plus the fact that I was thirty-eight years old, and I couldn't pick up my own kids. Didn't even have the strength left to keep them on my lap. That's no life for a man.

So when Dr. Kroner broached the idea to me by saying, "John, we don't know if you'll be taken as a candidate for surgery, but would you consider going out to Stanford University Medical Center, in California, and have them evaluate you for it?" I said yes. This was after Ann and I talked it over.

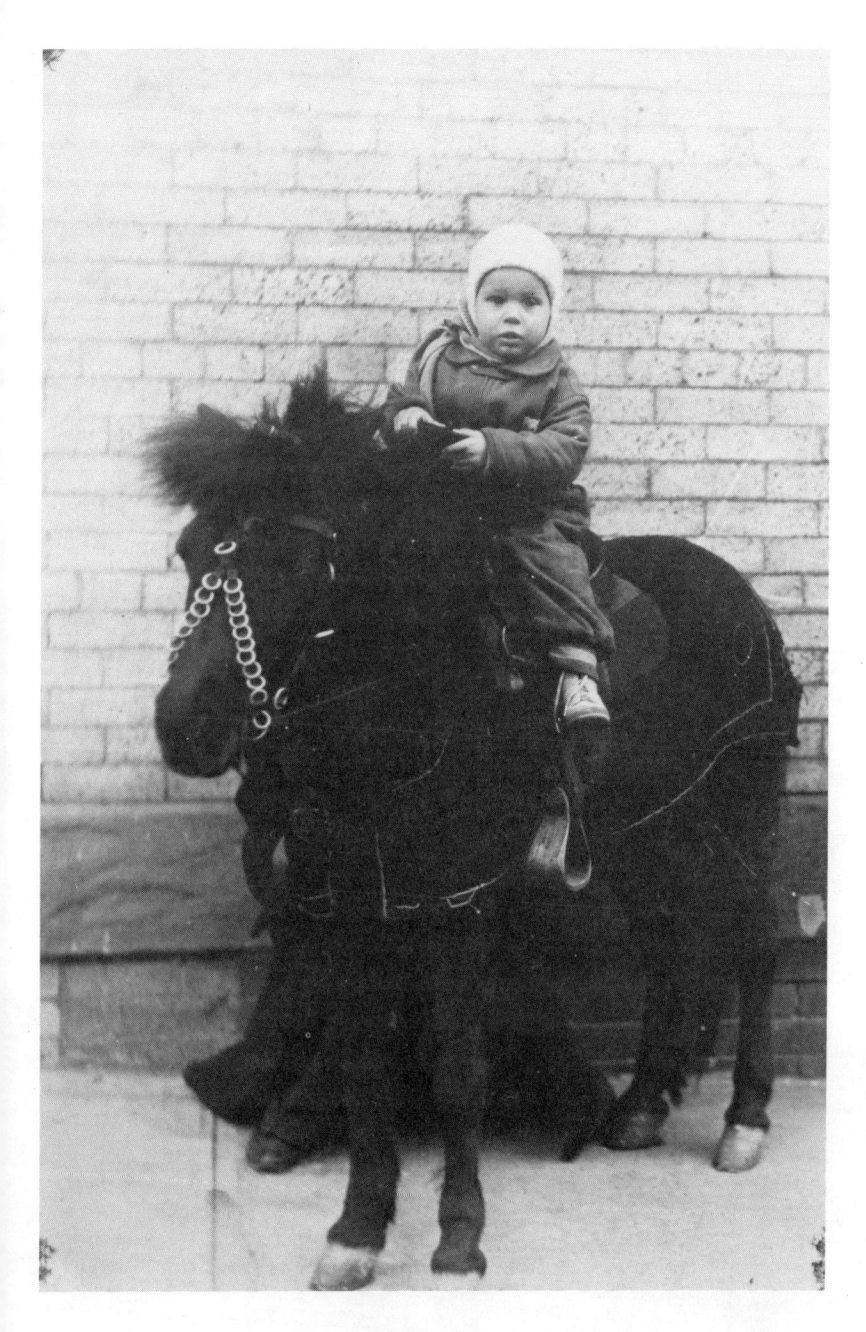

John, age two

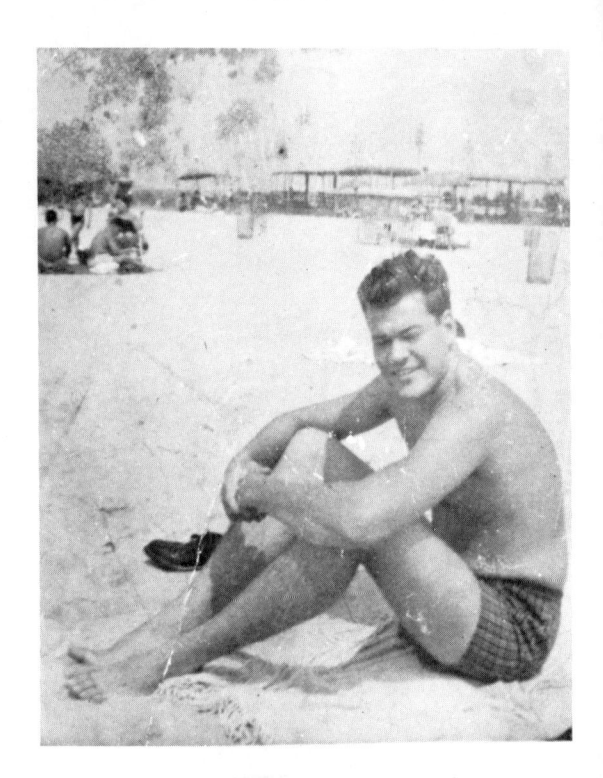

Rough and ready

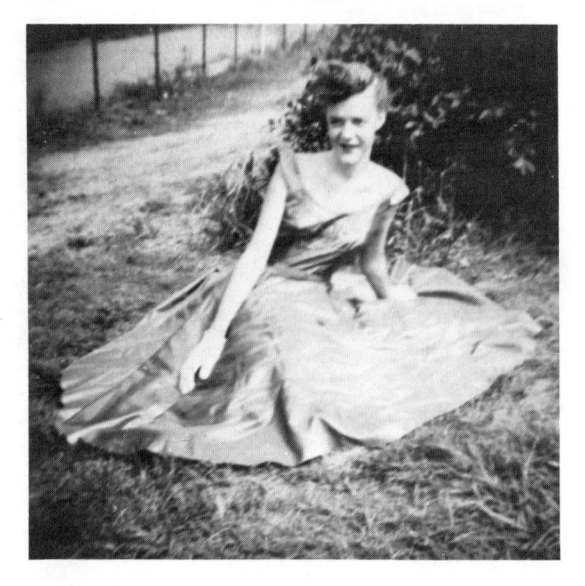

Sweet sixteen

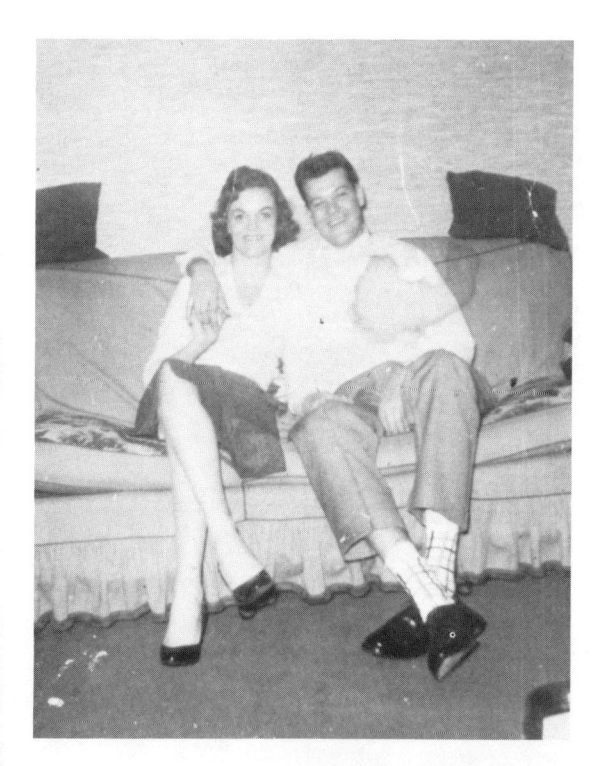

We're going steady

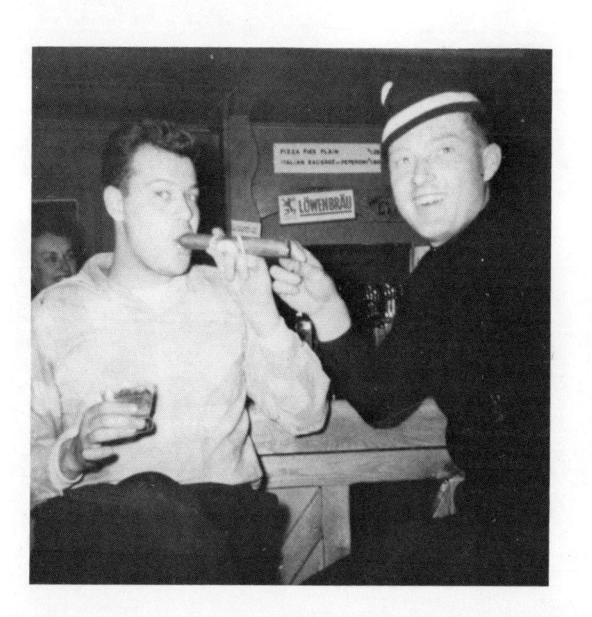

Double trouble

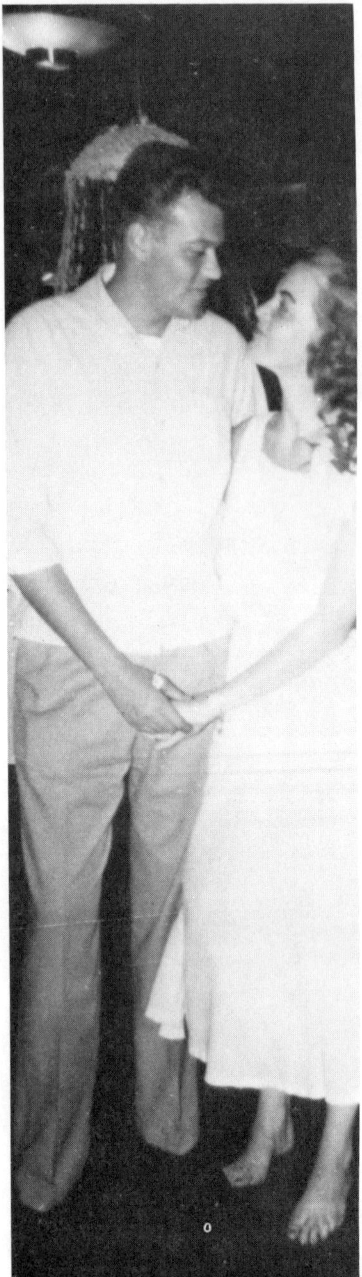

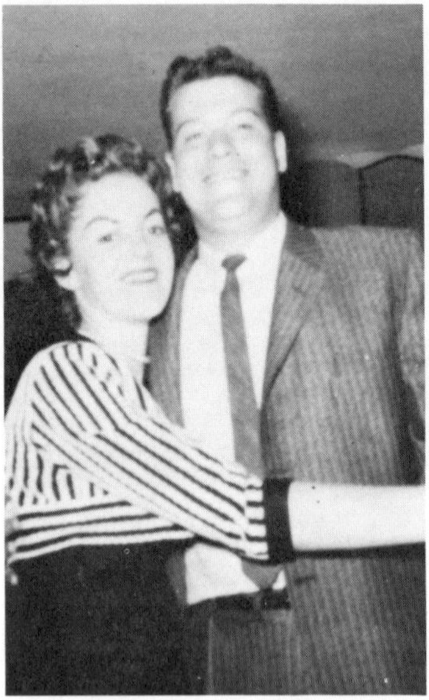

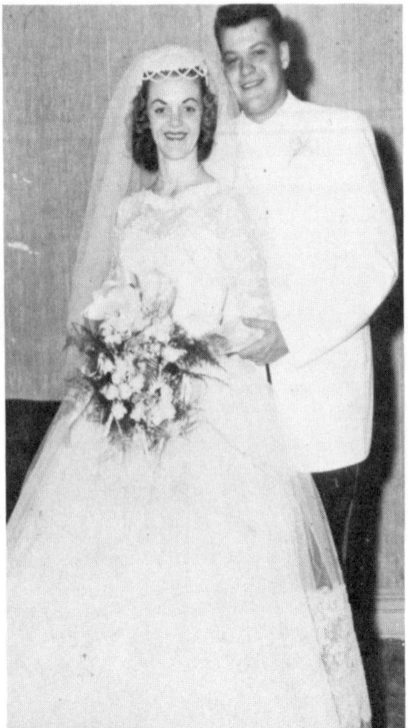

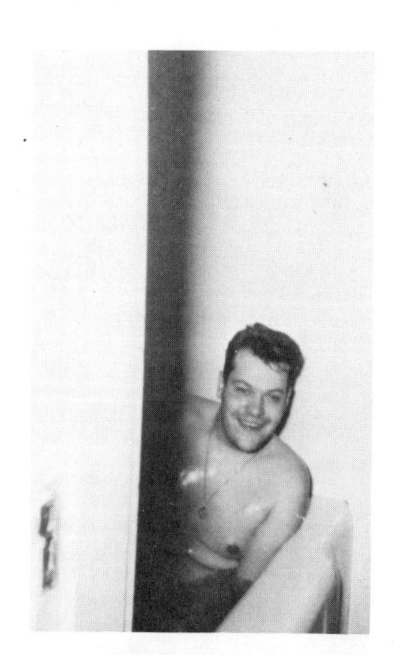

*Far left* Bridal shower, June 1957
*Above left* Oh, how we danced
*Below left* Just married
*Right* Time out
*Below* Daddy and baby Janice

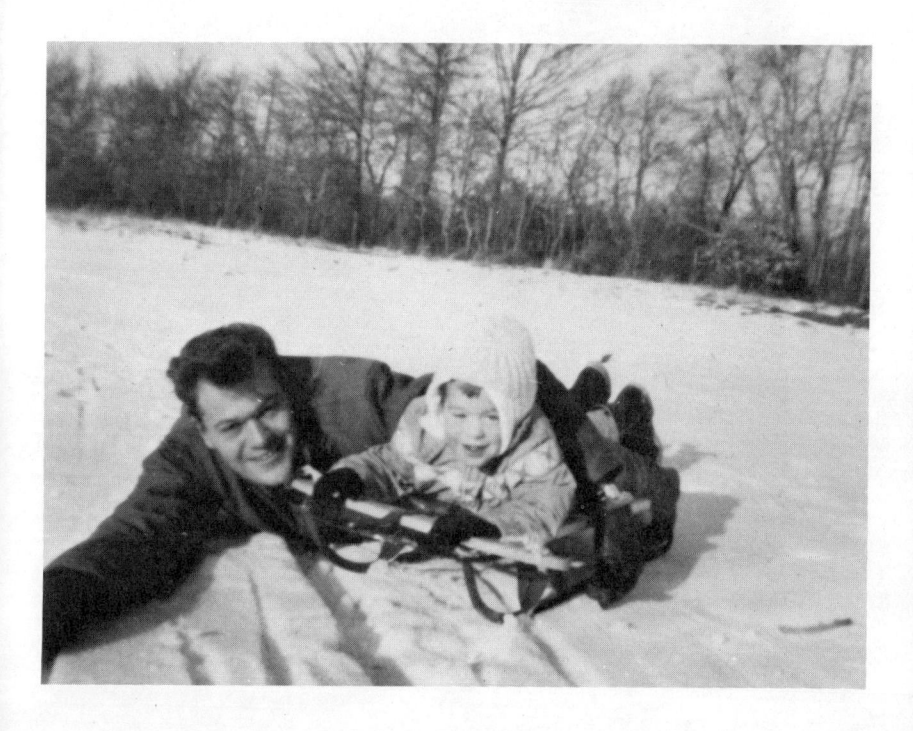

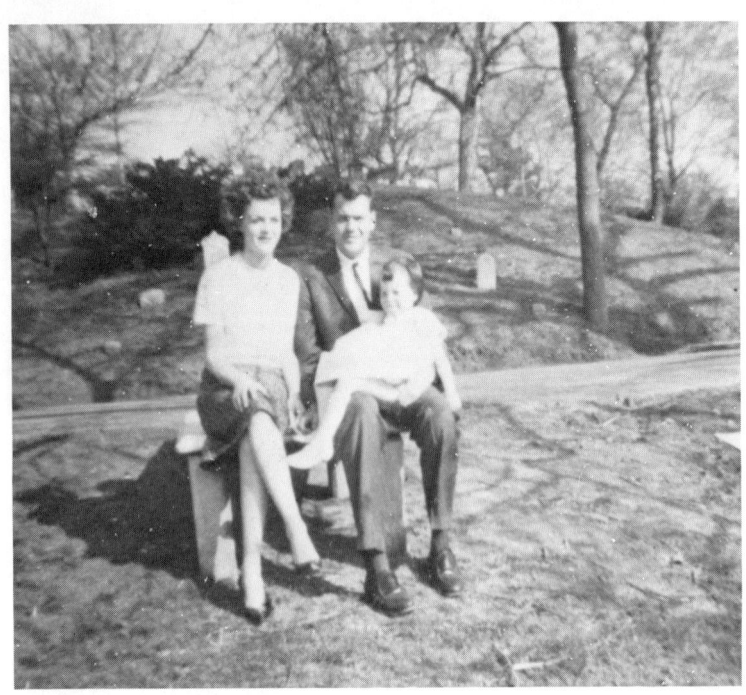

One Sunday afternoon

With Janice's snowman, "Ollie"

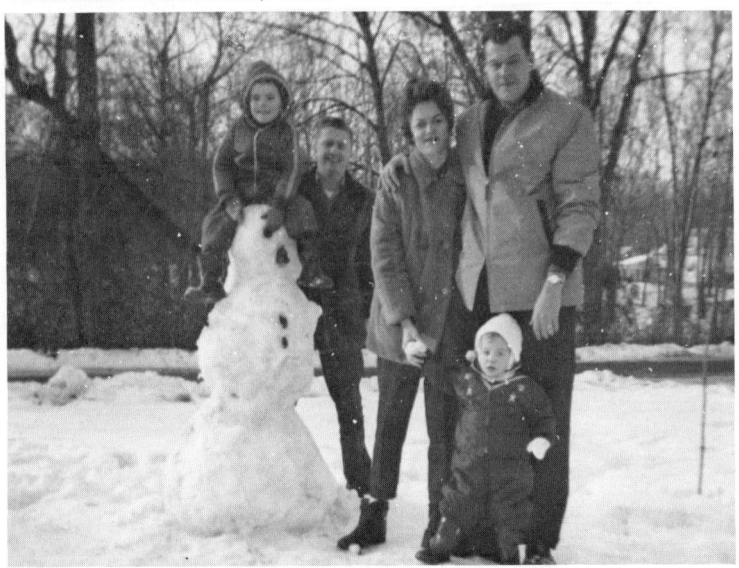

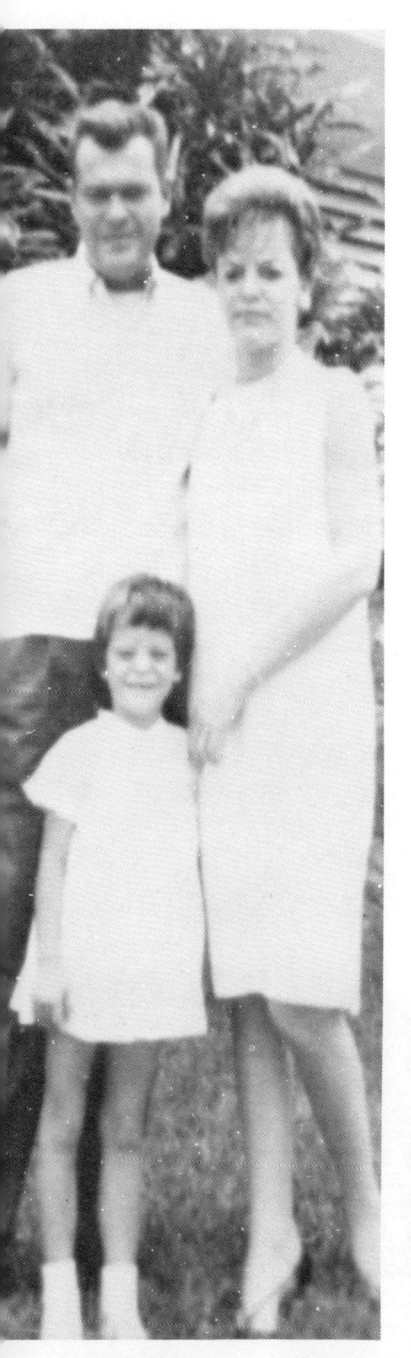

*Left* Puerto Rico, 1963

*Below* Janice and "Santa"

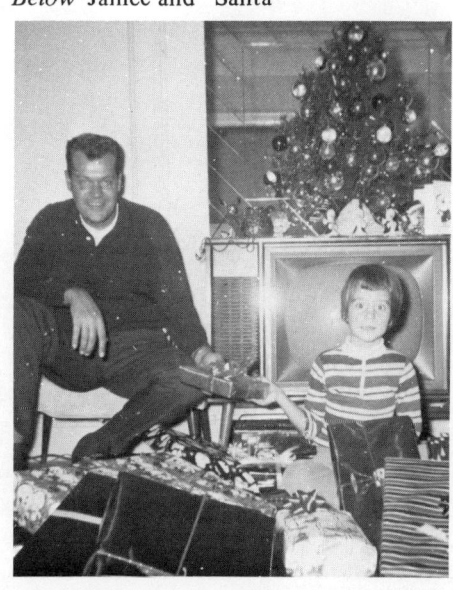

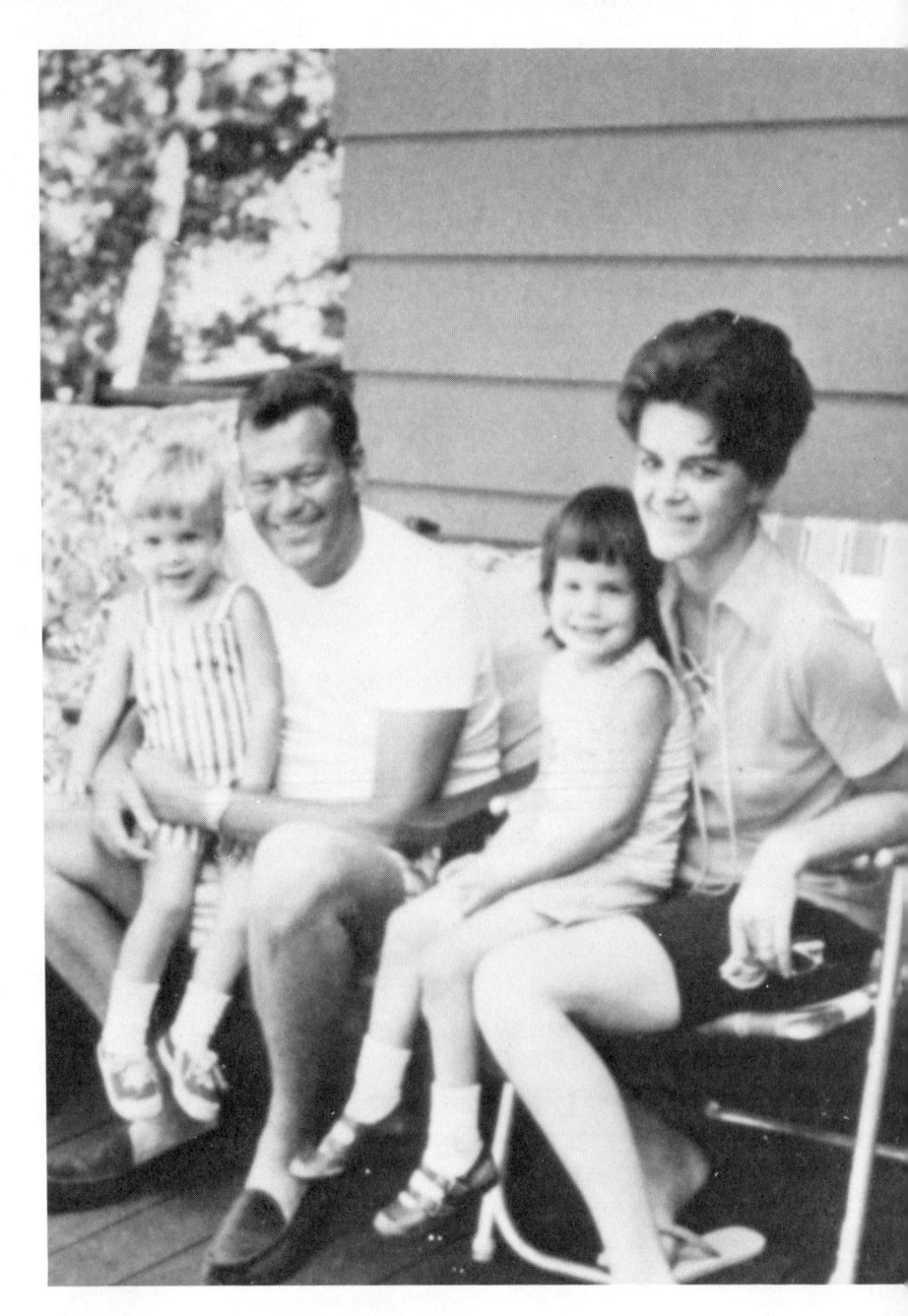

With Joanie and John Jr.

# TWO

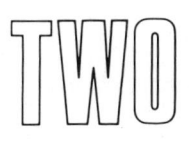

## TRANSPLANT

# 10

## Orders

*ANN* We came home from the hospital to wait for the call.

I began notifying the family, telling my parents, brothers, and sisters that Dr. Kroner was going to try and get him out to Stanford to be evaluated for a heart transplant. My mother started to cry. I heard her hand the phone to my father. He got on and didn't know what to say. He was very upset. He mumbled something about the good Lord, then said he'd have Mary call. My sister Mary. Mary called and asked if we needed money and what would happen to the children. Everybody called to find out if they could help out with money, running errands, or anything else.

Then we called John's sister, Joan. She was very encouraging and understanding. "You're doing the right thing. Both of you. It's the best thing to be done right now, and I know everything is going to be all right."

Then we called John's parents. I told them how bad John was.

But they just didn't want to believe it. I told them what we had decided to do. About the transplant idea.

His father said, "Don't have that done. Don't believe in it. Definitely not. I don't agree with it. It isn't safe enough yet."

His mother got on to say she didn't agree with it either.

I tried to make them understand, but I only made things worse. "Mom, Dad, you're hiding your heads in the sand. You feel that if you don't talk about something, it's just not there, or it'll probably go away. But John is in very serious shape. He *needs* this operation."

"Ann, don't have it done. Don't believe in it."

John got on and they wished him their love.

I woke up that night and found John just sitting in the chair that he smokes in, staring out the window. I didn't want to intrude. It was his own private thoughts. I went back to sleep. The next night, and the night after, he did the same thing. And this time I spoke to him.

"Are you afraid?"

"No. I'm really not. It's just that . . ."

"What? What is it?"

"I guess it's the fear of the unknown. Never mind. You go back to sleep."

"No. I want to talk to you. Tell me what's bothering you."

"It's just that . . . if anything happens . . ."

"Yes?"

"It's not that I'm asking . . ." He started to cry, and put his hands up to his eyes. "It's not that I'm asking you to promise not to marry again . . . or anything like that. That part of it doesn't bother me so much. But someone else . . . taking my place as the father of my *children*! Little John . . . my son . . . my wonderful son . . . after all the years of waiting for a son . . . and him calling somebody else . . . a stranger . . . *'Daddy.'* I guess that gets to me a little." I went over to him and kissed him. He put his head on my shoulder. "I know it's selfish of me, but the idea of you remarrying, and my children, who I'm never gonna get to know, calling somebody else . . . I know it's selfish of me. But I'll never see the little ones grow up. I'll never get to know them except as *babies*!"

Dr. Kroner called the next day. John took the call in the kitchen.

"John, you've got four days to get out to Stanford!"

"Four days? Hell! I was thinking of two or three weeks! We figured we would have at least two weeks to make plans and arrangements."

"Let me explain something to you. When Stanford Medical Center says they're ready to see you, you go when *they* say! If they get somebody else in the meantime, they may not take you at all. I've told them how much time you have left, and that it is literally a question of life or death. Fortunately, you've got a shot, because they have no other recipients waiting at the moment. So you go when *they* want you. Not when *you* want to!"

That afternoon we got a special delivery letter from Stanford, confirming our reservations. This was November 4, 1974. It said:

Dear Mr. Hurley:

This is to confirm that we are requesting a bed for you on the Stanford Cardiology Service on Saturday, Nov. 9, and cardiac catheterization studies have been scheduled for the 11th. This has been arranged for you by your physician, Dr. Kroner, through Dr. Schroeder of our Division.

If you feel you need an ambulance when you arrive at the airport, you can call Fields Ambulance Co., (415) 968–1616. They have both standard ambulance service and "care cab" (also known as "wheel chair service") available. (The wheel chair service involves driver and wheelchair only, no attendant, no gurney, and patient must be able to walk.) Taxis are of course available at the airport. I would suggest that you enter via the Emergency Entrance of the hospital, since that way you can be taken direct to your room, and your wife can then go to the admitting office and take care of admitting paperwork for you.

I am enclosing various maps and information leaflets for you, as well as a list of hotels and motels. To assist you in planning, the cost of living is fairly high in this area, and a bare minimum of $100 per week for one person should be allowed, or between $500–600 per month for two people. We suggest the family stay in temporary hotel or motel accommodation while the patient is being evaluated. Then in the event the patient is selected as a transplant candidate, they can make arrangements for an apartment.

The patient is responsible for payment of his hospital and medical expenses during the evaluation period and any inpatient or outpatient care prior to transplant surgery. (In the event transplant surgery does take place, there is grant assistance available from the time of actual surgery.) Please bring your insurance forms, with your portions filled out and signed, for the admitting office. (Since costs at this Center are high, you may wish to check with your insurance carrier as to extent of coverage relative to California prices, as well as to check on how much of your total benefits you have left available to you.)

It would be helpful if you could call and let me know your flight number and time of arrival. Meanwhile if you have any questions, please let me know. We understand you will bring medical records with you. Please be sure to include X-rays and any cineangiograms. Thank you.

> Sincerely,
>
> (Miss) H. Knott
> Cardiology Division
> Patient Representative

*JOHN* I hadn't thought at all about finances until I finished reading the letter from Stanford. I had virtually exhausted my savings. But I hadn't touched our stocks. I called my broker. The market was depressed as hell. We needed the cash. The airfare alone to California was costly for two people. And it damn well wasn't likely we were going to win the tickets on any quiz show in the near future. Plus Ann would have to be living in a motel. These are all expenses that you can't collect from an insurance company. This is strictly out of your own pocket. I had no choice but to sell at tremendous losses. I lost my ass. For example, I had 1000 shares of Diamondhead, worth $13,500. When I sold the stock, I got $1800. for it! Utter necessity. Nothing else to do. We needed the money.

Then Bobbie and Ronnie came to us. They wanted to help out any way they could, and offered to take the children while we were away.

I said to them, "You're gonna be taking an awful lot on yourself."

And they said, "No. No. We've talked it over, and we want to take the three children. In fact, we'd love to have them, and that's that. We don't want to break them up. Ronnie and I can never forget that when we were first moving up here, and we didn't have enough money for the down payment on the house ... if it hadn't been for you, John, with no strings attached, no interest ... and you coming forward to help us, we wouldn't have our house up here today."

So it was agreed to. I left a bankbook with them, to help pay for the children's expenses.


*ANN* The night before we left, some neighbors called. They wanted to come over and wish us luck. Carol and Frank Gonzalez, Rich and Jan Traeger, Howard and Joan Snizak, Jerry and Georgia Wood, Norene and Bernt, and Bobbie and Ronnie. We had a champagne party. John had won a case of champagne during the World Series. Inside of a few minutes we were having the time of our lives, laughing it up, clinking glasses, swapping jokes. Janice came in for a minute but saw how everyone was laughing it up, so she went back to her room. We pretty well finished off that case.

After everyone left, I put the glasses into the dishwasher. Then John and I sat down in the TV room. It was a letdown after the party. We both looked at each other and felt very emotional. Because as they were leaving, our friends had handed us several hundred dollars. Pressed it into our hands. We were deeply touched by this.

We went downstairs to the bedroom to pack. The phone rang. It was John's sister, Joan. "I've given Mom and Dad a lot of literature on transplants—how successful they are, and how much farther they've come up with it—and now they say it's OK to go ahead and be evaluated, and *have* the transplant. They've read up on it."

A few minutes later, John turned to me. "Would you call my parents? I want to talk to them before we go."

I reached them and didn't say much. "John wants to speak to both of you." And I handed him the phone.

His mother and father broke down on the phone. They wished him luck. But I could tell they were afraid for him. The conversation ended with John saying, "Let's hope everything turns out all right. Right, Dad. So long, Dad. So long, Mom."

The following morning (Saturday, November 9), Norene came to take the little ones while we were going out to the airport. Little John thought he was just going to stay for a little while at "Tanta's" house. But Joanie was another story. She realized that we were going away. So she hid from us. We had to go find her. She was hiding in the dining room, behind the drapes. I kept calling for her. "Joanie. Come on out, Joanie. Where are you,

Joanie?" And she didn't answer. You could see her little feet sticking out from under the curtain, and her little braid, also, and John said, "I found her! I found her! I see you!" And he's playing peek-a-boo with her!

But she just screamed and threw herself on the floor. She wasn't going to go. There was no walking her out, anyway. She was still holding on to her blanket all this time. She wanted to come with us. "Wanna go with Mommy! Go with Daddy! Wanna go with Mommy!"

So I took her aside and tried to reassure her. "Joanie, honey, Mommy and Daddy are coming back. We're coming back soon, my darling. We just have to go for a little while and get Daddy a new heart. So he won't be sick any more. Wouldn't you like that, sweetheart? For Daddy to feel all good again? So we'll only be gone for a short time, my angel. We won't be gone long. And we'll call you on the telephone lots of times, and send you letters, and you'll stay with your Aunt Bobbie and Uncle Ronnie, and Janice will be there with you, and you can help take care of your little baby brother."

This did absolutely no good whatsoever. She started crying again, even more than before. She was screaming, and she refused to budge. Norene picked her up, bodily, and took her out to the car, put her in the back seat, and locked the door. She already had baby John in his car seat, strapped in.

And for a brief moment, I didn't want to go either. It hit me that I was being separated from my babies, for how long I didn't know. And I didn't want to be away from them. But then I realized that there was absolutely no choice, no real choice, at all.

We had been notified to go out to Stanford on very short notice. I called up to make flight reservations on first class, and requested that there be extra oxygen on board in case there was a problem. Dr. Kroner suggested it, as a precaution.

The first airline I spoke to said this was impossible. They would not let us on board with extra oxygen. The reservation clerk I spoke to said, "If he's that sick, he shouldn't be flying." I said "Goddamn it! If he wasn't sick I wouldn't be taking him out to California for a heart transplant!" And she said, "I really don't think you can take him on board without some kind of certificate, like a medical OK, and a doctor accompanying him. I'll have to check with our medical department." So I asked to speak to her supervisor. He gets on and says, "Mrs. Hurley, we haven't ever heard of taking extra oxygen on board, but if your doctor writes to our doctor and explains the situation, we most probably can work it out. It just has to go through the proper channels. You understand. But in any event, we have nothing leaving Newark Airport at the time you've requested. May I suggest you check with another airline?"

My neighbor Jan Traeger heard about the problem we were having booking a flight, and fortunately she had relatives who worked for United Airlines. She called them and explained there was a medical emergency, and that John was going out for a possible heart transplant, and got us the reservations with the extra oxygen. But on such short notice that they had to bump someone.

United had a wheelchair waiting for us at Newark Airport and took us into the VIP lounge and served us coffee while we all said our good-byes. Jim and Jean Clark and their twelve-year-old-son Dana were there. My sister Barbara and brother-in-law Ronnie. And Janice. We all got very emotional. John asked Jim and Bobbie and Ronnie to take care of us, his family, if anything happened to him. And they told him not to worry about anything. That they would definitely take care of everybody. My sister said, "John. Please stop worrying. You'll be back. You've been through so much already—you *have* to be back."

Then John got very serious and turned to Jim. "Jim. I'm counting on you. You know everybody at work as far as insurance is concerned. And if something does happen, I want you to coordinate everything with Ann to make sure everything is taken care of." He handed Jim a typed piece of paper. "Here's a list of where my life insurance policies are, what debts I owe, what stock options I've collateralized through the bank, and everything else you'll need to know to take care of Ann's financial interests."

"Don't worry about it, John. Everything will be taken care of."

We had been told by a steward that we could all board the plane and say our good-byes there before they took off. So we all went to the gate, and everybody started to go up the ramp. And there was a slight snafu. The flight steward comes over to us.

"I'm sorry. The family has to leave. There's been a change in the schedule, and we're running behind. Everybody has to leave, and you'll have to board now."

Janice looked stricken. She hadn't said two words during the whole day. And now she had to be parted from us. She started crying, then she threw her arms around her father. "Oh Daddy! Please be well. Please be all right. I'm praying for you."

"Thank you, sweetheart. I will. I will."

Everybody was getting emotional now. I embraced Janice and held her close. "I'll bring Daddy back. Don't you worry. I promise you. He's going to be back, and he'll be just fine, and we'll all be together again."

The steward was almost pushing us on the plane now, to keep to his schedule. He wanted to avoid the rush of the crowd that was about to descend on us. We look back. I can see my sister, and Jim and Jean, and even their son, their eyes all filling up. John was crying now too. He managed a slight wave of good-bye. And very softly he said, "God bless you all."

The airline had been really efficient. When we got on board, there was this huge oxygen tank underneath our seat. People kept looking at it for the whole trip, like it was a bomb or something. It was four feet long and a foot and a half in diameter. And it took the whole space under the two seats we were sitting on. And there were signs placed all around us which said, "NO SMOKING. DANGER. OXYGEN. NO SMOKING!" People kept whispering, "What's going on?"

Suddenly, we hear this woman screaming. Like a shrew. "Who the hell took my seat? I had reservations booked three months ago! My husband booked our reservations last August! Dammit! Dammit to hell!" It was the woman we had bumped! John and I just put our heads down and didn't say a word. You wouldn't believe the screaming that went on in that plane!

The woman looked like money. She not only looked it, she expressed herself as being from money as well. She collared the flight steward. "I want you to know that my husband and I have traveled all over the world and are consistent customers of United Airlines, and just what the hell is going *on* here? We had confirmed reservations months ago!" She was traveling with her husband, who I immediately recognized as a leading man, an actor on one of the daytime soap operas. And the reason she was screaming so loudly was that now only *one* of them was going to be allowed in the first class section! And needless to say, *he* wasn't going to give up *his* seat! He was a *STAR*! So she was furious. *Ranting. She* was going to have to go *tourist*!

# 11

## Stanford University Medical Center

*JOHN*  We got out to California, and I was *smashed*.

The last thing I did before leaving was ask the doctor if I could have a couple of drinks on the plane. "No problem, John. Have as many as they'll give you." So I did. And I was taking quite a bit of Valium as well, so I was really feeling no pain. So I had a couple of martinis. And champagne. It was a champagne flight. Then I had some wine with my meal. And an after-dinner drink. Anything they would give me. This was gonna be a flight to remember! And a martini after that!

Our friends Jackie and Mike Ladner were waiting for us at the airport. Jackie is an ex-nun who dropped out of the convent. She's got reddish hair, is in her early thirties, wears dark horn-rimmed glasses, and has nice brown eyes. Mike worked with me in Puerto Rico as a special commodities manager for the Caribbean area, so at one time indirectly worked for me. When we get off the plane, I see he's wearing cowboy boots, a Western shirt, wide leather belt and buckle, and looks like Roy Rogers himself.

I tried to get Mike to stop off for another drink before we checked into the hospital. Nothing doing. He was like an expectant father. Jackie told us, "Mike practiced the fastest route to the hospital—to find the quickest way to get you there." I said, "I believe it." He refused to stop anywhere. So we went straight to the hospital. There's such a thing as stretching loyalty too far!

They wheeled me in through the emergency entrance 'round the back, as the letter from Stanford instructed us to do. This section was completely under construction at that time. And my first impression of the place was, My God! What kind of a *dump* is this? There were walls knocked out, canvas drapes hanging down, scaffolding all around. It looked like where they might dump the garbage! It was terrible! Rags. Paint cans. Newspapers. Ladders. "This doesn't look like no hospital to me! It looks more like a shit house!" And Jackie's saying "The front of it looks nice, Ann. It really does. It really looks nice out front."

It's really a gorgeous hospital. The grounds are breathtaking. If we'd been admitted through the front, I'd have seen the fountain, which lights up at night, and the sculptured lawns and gardens. But I didn't see any of that that day. They wheeled me through these underground subterranean passages, and all the time I'm saying to myself, *What* the hell kind of a hospital *is* this? Could they do the transplants *here*? God *forbid*! It looks more like a meat packing plant!

The plane had landed at 1:00 in the afternoon, and by 2:30 I had already had an EKG. At 3:00 I had chest X-rays, and at 4:00 they gave me a blood workup. The rush was on.

They put me in a ward with other people. Different people with different problems, mostly heart-related. The Medical Director of Cardiology was Dr. Schroeder. He came in to greet me, while a nurse was taking blood out of my arm. We shook hands —between syringes—and I explained to him that Dr. Kroner had asked me to correspond with him, and I had come up with the idea of keeping a small journal or diary of what was happening to me daily during my stay at Stanford.

"I'm going to keep a record of every test I'm given, and what time of day it's given on. If that's all right with you."

"That sounds like a fine idea. You're going to be directly involved, anyway."

*ANN* As soon as John came on the ward, they had a team of doctors come in and they didn't lose any time. They took blood, blood pressure, had an EKG taken. Started their tests. That's when Dr. Goodson came out into the hall to ask me a question.

"Mrs. Hurley. Please don't be offended by what I'm about to ask you. But believe me, I have only your husband's best interest in mind."

"What is it, Doctor?"

"Has your husband . . . has John ever talked about . . . or contemplated . . . *suicide*?"

I was shocked by his question. Really taken aback. Dr. Goodson was an intern, a very young guy, very tall and good looking. And when he came out of the room, I had been with Jackie and Mike, and he asked them to excuse us. He had some questions to ask me. He took me off to one side, and when he said that, I was really quite surprised at his impertinence.

"Why would you ask me that, Doctor?"

"Because . . . frankly, Mrs. Hurley, your husband seems extremely down . . . and very depressed."

"It's not what you think. John is just wrecked from the flight. He had a great deal to drink on the plane. He was very nervous about coming out here. And he's on tranquilizers, to boot. He takes quite a bit of Valium. And also, I think he's unhappy to be away from the children."

"He's on Valium?
"Yes."
"How much?"
"I think he takes forty milligrams a day."
"You're sure you're telling me everything? He's never attempted suicide?"
"Doctor Goodson! Please!"
"No offense, Mrs. Hurley. I'm just trying to do my job."
"I'll tell you . . . he *did* once say . . . that if he were to ever become a vegetable . . . and be forever lying in bed, helpless, not able to take care of himself . . . that he might take his own life."
"Did he ever tell you that he knew how?"
"Come to think of it, he did say once that if it came right down to it, there'd be an 'accident.' He'd be cleaning his rifle. But I don't think he ever would do it. I'm sure of it."
"Thank you, Mrs. Hurley."

A few minutes later, Mike Ladner, seeing all the people in this ward with John, says, "Sea-Land pays for private rooms. Why did they put John on a *ward*? I don't get this at all. What do you suppose is going on? Maybe we should talk to someone about this?"

"I don't know, Mike. But I don't think I should rock the boat. Especially not before the doctors give us any evaluation—and say whether they want to operate on John or not."

"Ann, John is a Sea-Land executive. I think we should march straight back to this chief doctor or whoever is in charge here and have him put John into a private room. I really do."

I got upset. But then I realized that Mike was so upset himself, he was talking out of nervousness and concern for John.

At 10:00 that night we had to leave John at the hospital. I kissed him good-night. "Good-night, babe, Everything's gonna be all right. Mike's taking Jackie and me out for something to eat. Then we're gonna check into the Holiday Inn. Jackie's staying the night with me. Then tomorrow, Mike's coming back to take us to church."

"Good-night, Ann. I'll see ya tomorrow."

*JOHN* Sunday, November 10th, was the following day. I had some skin patch tests at 10:00 a.m., to see if I was allergic to anything. Then at 11:00 I had another blood workup.

*Monday, November 11th.* I had my cardiac catheterization at 1:00 p.m. This is a three to four hour type of a thing. The catheterization involves going into a vein on your arm, and they feed a catheter up into your heart—and they use this to examine your coronary arteries, and each of the chambers of your heart. From the inside. Two tubes are actually fed in. One is for dye, which they actually inject, and the other has sort of a light on the end of it, so when they inject the dye they're taking videotape pictures of it, to find out how extensive the damage might be. This was the second time this kind of thing was done on me. The first one was exactly two years prior, to the exact day—at Beth Israel Hospital. When they had given me two years, on the outside, to live.

*Tuesday, November 12th.* I had an EKG at 10:00 a.m. a skull X-ray at 11:00, a thyroid scan, where they inject you with radioactive isotopes, at 2:00, a pulmonary function test at 4:00, and blood workups at 7:00 that night! You were going!

Eating was the biggest problem. Some days you ate, and some days you missed your lunch, or you'd come back and your food would be all cold; it would be laying there for two or three hours and nobody would take it out and keep it someplace.

By this time I was feeling lightheaded.

They gave me a glucose tolerance test to find out if I was diabetic. On the contrary, they found I had hypoglycemia. After that, they fed me small meals, six times a day. Bear in mind, they're wheeling me all around the hospital to take these tests.

*Wednesday, November 13th.* I had a liver scan at 11:00 a.m., an electroencephalogram at 1:30, and another blood workup at 4:00.

*Thursday, November 14th.* I had a lung scan, some more pulmonary function tests, and *another* blood workup at 4:00.

*Friday, November 15th.* I had a phonocardiogram at 10:00 a.m., an echocardiogram at 10:30, a blood workup at 12:00—and then one of my ears pierced! So help me! By a nurse who looked like a little dark gypsy!

I was in a ward with eight guys in this one room. They were running tests on all of us. There was this one guy, he was in his seventies, but he looked like one of the pioneers who originally rode out West. Real John Wayne type. Rough tough guy. You wouldn't mess with him. He had a cancer of some sort behind his ear, eating away at the bone. Now Stanford is a teaching hospital, and they have a lot of interns, and students, and residents. So every time they would come in to examine this guy, a troop of fifteen white coats would come marching in behind the chief doctor, and as soon as he saw them, he'd bellow, "Goddamn it! What the hell do you clowns want from me now? That goddamn Cox's Army is here again! Dammit to hell! Drat!"

There was another guy there, who was a hiring boss with the longshoremen. He was black. But you'd never know it from his outward appearance. He looked pure white—like Ivory Snow. Then one day his family came up to visit him. And in they walk. *The whole tribe, super black!* I couldn't believe it. Everybody on that ward did a double take. And he had a daughter who was the most absolutely gorgeous colored girl I have *ever* seen. Took my breath away. Which under the circumstances wasn't hard to do!

We had one guy who was a fire chief. They thought he had just had a heart attack, so they were running tests on him. I later became friendly with him.

Then there was this real old guy who was terminal. He was located between Cox's Army and the fire chief. Now *this* guy really did it to us! There were two TVs in the room, facing in opposite directions. So if I was sitting on one side, I could look across, while laying in bed, at the TV facing me. Likewise with the other patients on the opposite side of the room. They would be looking at the TV that was directly over *my* head. The TV *I* watched was over the *old* guy's head. *Comprende?*

Now here's where the problem was. The old guy, who was in his late eighties and used to sleep all day—he was very tall and thin with a face like a chicken hawk—he was a bit confused. So at night, after we'd all run the gantlet of tests, we'd be interested in a ball game or good cop show, and the four of us on the one side were looking at the TV that was over *his* head. So what he'd do is—he'd get *out* of bed, come over to *our* side, and without any warning whatsoever, he'd take our little remote control thing and change the picture that all four of us are sittin' there in the middle of watching! No questions. Just *CLICK*! And we'd be sittin' there watching cartoons! He thought it was *his* TV, because it was over *his* bed, on *his* side of the room! On top of that, he was very hard of hearing, and he'd turn the sound up so it was *blasting*. Maybe he was senile. I don't know. But he'd just get up out of bed, and everybody's watching a ball game, and all of a sudden we're watching Bugs Bunny! Or Woody Woodpecker!

To me it was hysterical. There we were, a room full of heart patients all trying to remain calm, and he's playing hob with our knob!

One of the nurses who was up there on this ward was a real tough top-sergeant type of woman. If she wasn't ex-Marine

Corps, she sure looked and sounded like it. She was stocky, maybe 5'6" and heavy set. Must have been in her forties. Reminded me of Broderick Crawford in drag. She had no sympathy for anybody. But she was as good as gold. She wouldn't take any crap from anybody. For instance, when some of the other nurses were on, we could sneak a cigarette or two. But when she was on, there was NO SMOKING, period. She'd take whatever we were using for ashtrays, usually paper cups, and go around putting water in 'em! Not so subtle. "Just making sure you don't start any fires, boys." I started calling her Sergeant Nurse.

For some reason she had something against this transplant of mine. Toward the middle of this week of tests, she kept repeating to Ann and me, "Are you sure you people know what you're doing?"

Ann looks at her and says, "I hope *they* know what they're doing!"

And she says "Well, I'd sure as heck never let 'em give a transplant to me."

And I say, "I think that should be up to the doctors."

And she keeps right on going. "Do you know they're actually going to *kill* you? For at least ninety minutes?"

Ann gulps and says, "Whattaya mean they kill him for ninety minutes? What in hell are you talking about?"

I guess you just don't stop and think they *are* going to "kill you," in a sense. They take your heart out while you're on the heart-lung machine, and then they take the donor's heart and sew it into your chest! But the way she blurts the whole thing out, it scared the bejeezus out of us. I think we should have reported it. We never did. But I'm sure she would've frightened anybody who was on the borderline into maybe backing out. She didn't mean any harm from it. She was just saying what was on her mind, and letting the chips fall.

This whole week I was writing my journal for Dr. Kroner. On paper towels and napkins! I was wearing a bathrobe as they wheeled me from one test area to another, and I scribbled my notes with a ball point pen and stuffed them into my pockets. I later mailed them to Dr. Kroner. Each night before I went to sleep, I prepared the envelope for mailing.

I remember writing on one napkin, "Hey, Doc! Maybe I'm just paranoid, but I'm starting to get a funny feeling about these guys in the white jackets!"

They also had some pretty fancy gadgets they fitted me with. One was a wireless transmitter that sent my heart pulses to a monitor in my room. This way my heart was always being monitored no matter where I was in the hospital. Pretty neat.

They have "messenger boys," they call them, who wheel you around the hospital for the tests, to wherever the next test is being performed. One morning I ran out of cigarettes, and I had been having at least three a day, despite the doctor's prohibition. So the messenger drops me outside where they're gonna do this thyroid scan, and I'm waiting my turn. This old gent is sitting across from me, also in a wheelchair.

I started talking to him. He was in his sixties, built very heavy, with very gray hair and faded eyes. But he looked like a nice guy. And he was telling me he was part of a group of twenty veterans that were brought over from the VA hospital, who all had throat cancer. He had already had his larynx removed and was speaking by this new way of talking by actually belching. It's really quite effective. So I tell him, "By the way, my wife will be late today. And I can't buy any cigarettes in the hospital. Can I bum one from you?"

And with this, he opens his bathrobe, and he's got a pack of menthol cigarettes in his shirt pocket, and a pack of regular in his bathrobe pocket!

"Which kind do you prefer?" This guy has just had his larynx removed! "Menthol or regular?"

"Regular would be just fine, thank you."

He gives me the whole pack! So of course I was set for the week. Great man! A delightful man.

# 12

## Psychological Tests

*ANN*  Before John was accepted as a candidate for the transplant program, we both had to take a number of psychological tests. They were trying to find out if both of us could *emotionally* accept the tremendous change that getting a new heart would bring.

We were interviewed by a woman. She was in her forties, had a very pleasant face, was petite, thin, and blonde. I'm not sure if she was a psychologist, or psychiatrist, or a psychiatric social worker. She was charming. But always very professional. She asked us to call her Sylvia. At first we met in her office. She told us she would try to answer any questions we had.

John started out by asking about other heart transplant patients. How many had died. How long he *really* had to live. And what the operation would cost. That's all he kept hammering away at was the cost of the operation. And what his chances were. But from the time he'd come to the hospital, I don't think he really ever actually *believed* he was really going to get a heart transplant. He felt certain that, at the last minute, the doctors would find something that could be mended. Like an artery or something. Or a valve. He would just not accept the fact that he might possibly be accepted for a transplant.

Sylvia explained to us that financial considerations were the last thing Stanford Medical Center worried about. The staff just wanted to know for sure that he and I were stable enough and intelligent enough to adapt and adjust to this new change in our lives if they did go ahead and perform the transplant. She told us that apparently it was a tremendous emotional strain on some people. She cited one example, a young man who could not—emotionally—accept the fact that he actually had another person's heart beating inside his chest. She told us that they almost lost him completely after the operation, because of his severe depression. He had come through the surgery beautifully and was going along with no problems, no rejection—and all of a sudden he started walking the hallways with his head down, in complete despair.

He was a zoo-keeper by profession. Same age as John. And they told him that he would not be able to return to his job, because of the danger of infection. He knew this going in. We used to see him walking the halls. He was very thin, exceptionally so, with hippy long brown hair that hung below his shoulder blades. We knew who she was talking about. Finally, she told us, he just stopped walking the hallways. And just wanted to die, his depression was so deep. He just refused to accept the fact that he had someone else's heart beating inside him, and that he wouldn't be able to have his old job back. He felt he'd rather be dead, after all.

Sylvia admitted to us, "He could be one of the fellas we made a mistake on." That's why they wanted to be sure we'd both mentally accept it. Because if you don't, you've lost the whole shooting match.

She also explained that they wanted to be sure that we didn't have any religious or other hangups which might prevent us from accepting a new heart. It's all so experimental, she told us, that they're learning, themselves, all the time.

We had long conversations. Almost every day. We talked in her office, in the cafeteria, in the hallways, in John's room, and in the conference room. Sometimes John and I were together. Sometimes she spoke to us separately. At first, our defenses were up. We felt we were on trial. So we were on our best behavior. Afraid of saying the wrong thing. Or possibly making a Freudian slip of some kind. Something that would put us out of the running.

That's when I realized that John, deep down, *knew* he had to have this operation, to *survive*. And that by not letting himself believe he was going to actually get a new heart, he was blocking his true feelings. In case they turned him down. I think he dreaded that possibility. I know I did.

*JOHN* The first time we talked, it was a little tense. We were in Sylvia's office. She started it off with a general kind of question, like, "Tell me a little about yourself," and I fidgeted in my chair for a second or two, thinking of what to say.

"Well. Before I came out to California, I was the vice-chairman of the planning board for Byram Township in New Jersey. Where we come from. We reviewed site plans, subdivisions, and master plans, to make sure that the builders complied with our local ordinances and standards. They're holding the seat open for me right now, until I get back. I was appointed by the mayor. Before that I was Director of Special Commodities for Sea-Land Service. That's a division of R.J. Reynolds."

Sylvia made a few notes. "Sounds very interesting. But I'm more interested in you. I mean, as a *person,* rather than what you've done. For example, are there any hobbies or other special interests that you enjoy?"

"Hobbies? Well . . . before my heart attack I was strictly an outdoorsman. I liked to hunt and fish. The lake where we live is stocked with trout, bass, pickerel, wall-eye, blue gills, and catfish. And perch. I take 'em home and clean 'em, and we have 'em for dinner. Had my Garcia pole and reel for ten years now. Same with my Ithaca twelve-gauge shotgun. I also have a Remington twenty-two. We go hunting for rabbits, pheasant, and deer. I belong to a gun club."

"Does Ann enjoy the same things you do?"

"Maybe she should answer that. No. Ann doesn't like to get involved with any of the wild game I bring home. So I clean the rabbits and pheasants myself, right in the kitchen sink. The kids usually come in and want to play with the feathers. When we first moved up to Forest Lakes, we had deer right on our front lawn.

I go hunting within walking distance of the house. It would be the equivalent of ten blocks away. You have to find a place to hide behind. Like a tree or a boulder. And be very quiet. And you just wait for a deer to come by. I aim for the head or heart area. Then after you bring 'em down, you dress 'em right out there. Gut 'em, so that when you get it home, it's all cleaned already."

I kept wondering if Sylvia might take this the wrong way, but I kept right on going.

"You take all their insides out, the guts and the entrails. The racoons take care of what you leave behind. Then you put it on the car and drive home with it. I hang it from a tree, right outside the kitchen window. For about a week. To let the meat age. In the morning, when everybody gets up for breakfast, Ann looks outside and always goes nuts! The deer, with his tongue hanging out of the side of his mouth—that's just what she wants to see in the morning!"

I paused and looked at Sylvia. She had a very neutral look on her face, and said, "I can imagine."

"Then, after it's aged, you take it to a butcher, who cuts, wraps, and freezes it for you. You can wind up with seventy-five to a hundred pounds of meat. To me, it's a good sport. Those deer are a hell of a lot smarter and faster than you think they are! I remember the first deer that I ever bagged. Pardon me for saying this—but I shot him in the *ass*!"

I thought Ann was going to die. She tried to sink down deep into her seat.

"I spotted him, and he was on the run, and I shot him, and he went down, and I ran like hell over to him and put him away with a second shot. In the head."

Sylvia just said, "Hmmmm." Then she said, "Tell me, John. Why do you suppose you had a heart attack in the first place? Why do you think it happened to *you*? After all, you're such a young man."

"I've given that a lot of thought. And . . . well . . . I guess I feel that God has a list. I feel that everybody, regardless of who they are, has a time and a date when their destiny is doomed. And when that time comes, you're gonna go. That's why you'll see innocent people walking across a street, and BOOM! They get hit by a truck. And that's *it*. I just feel that their number was up at that time."

I was perspiring and drying the palms of my hands on my pants. All Sylvia said was, "That's very interesting."

"We're all part of a Grand Design. Wars, hurricanes, earthquakes, things that wipe people out. It's His means of reducing populations. If you were to take all the people that were killed in major disasters and major wars and put them all here in the U.S.A., what would you have? You'd have one hell of a food problem! That's right! So I think it's Nature. And Nature itself automatically reverts back to God."

Sylvia nodded as if to say she understood what I was saying.

"And all of the assassinations, too. *All* of us have a time when it's gonna happen. And when that time comes, regardless of what you're gonna do, you've gotta go. And there's no way of getting out of it."

She nodded and wrote something down. Then she said, "OK, here's a question on an entirely different subject."

"Go ahead."

"Do you have any pet hate? Or, to put it another way, what do you hate the most? This can be anything or anyone. A person, a car, a political party, taxes. Anything. Like for example, what do you hate the most about your heart condition?"

"Well, you're limited. You can't really do what you'd like to do all the time. That sort of gets to me. God forbid I should have a flat tire someplace! And other things, too. Just before we came out here, Ann bought a new jar of peanut butter. And so help me, I didn't have the strength to open it by myself. I had to get Ann to do it."

"How did you feel about that?"

"How do you *think* I felt? I felt goddamn angry about it."

*ANN* She made some more notes. John and I looked at each other. We were wondering how we were doing. We couldn't tell. After a while Sylvia looked up from her scribbling.

"Tell me a little about yourself, Ann. Do you work?"

"No, I don't. John won't let me work. He won't let me find a job, to help out. He's *never* permitted me to work. Those children were never to be left alone. Many times I wanted to go back to work when Janice, our oldest, was ten or eleven, and I wasn't expecting. But there was no way. And we didn't need the money. John was making a very good salary. I just wanted to keep busy. But he often said that he had working parents, and he came home to an empty house. And he didn't like it."

Then she turned to John and asked how he felt about what I'd said, and I remember his very words. He said, "I don't believe in a mother not being home when the kids come home. But I was too young to really remember much of my own childhood.

I can remember Joan and I both had our chores to do, every day. We'd peel the potatoes, and put them in water, and place the pots on the stove so when my mother came home, she'd turn on all the burners and we'd have supper. And lunch time, we had to come home and fix our own lunches. We didn't live that far from school. So *I want my wife to be at home* when the kids come home from school. There's no question about it. Nothing even to discuss."

Then she asked me what *my* parents were like.

"Anna and Joseph? My mother and father fight to this day! She's hard of hearing but she doesn't admit it. They've been fighting for forty-eight years. My mother curses like a truck driver—but she's never had a sick day in her life. I swear, this has relieved all their tension—because they love each other very very deeply, and they'd do anything for each other. They've never left each other's side."

She wrote something down.

"And this may sound funny, but my mother never had a 'social' day out until her children were all off and married. *She was never out of her housedress!*"

Sylvia smiled.

"Never in her *life*! Until we were all gone! Five girls and two boys. She was a typical mother, I guess. But it's interesting, now that we're all raised, my mother is a *totally* different woman. She goes on the town every weekend. They socialize constantly. Before we were out and married, though—and I really mean this —the only function I ever saw that woman get dressed up for and leave the house for was the annual Railroad Dance. My father was a brakeman, a switcher, working for the railroad at Bush Terminal. And once a year they would have a Railroad Dance. In New York. At the Waldorf Astoria. Once a year. That's the only time I remember seeing her dressed up!"

"You refer to your mother as a 'typical' mother. Do you think of yourself that same way?"

"Someone once said—about five years ago, before John's heart attack—that I'm constantly cleaning or constantly in the house, and that I'm *just* a dedicated mother and wife. One of those 'types.' And I resented that. I said, 'Whattaya mean *type*?' And she says, 'One of those lackeys who are constantly on their knees in the house, taking care of the kids and taking care of your husband.' Well, I told her, 'I don't feel that I'm a lackey. I feel that this is my *job* in life. I love John, I love my children, and I love doing it. *And* taking care of the house.' I think John feels more tied down now that the little ones are here. There's ten years between Janice and Joanie. So he feels more tied down with three, rather than with one."

"Do the two of you fight over money?"

"Are you kidding? Our money fights? Hah! While he was still working—it was probably our biggest battle! Where did it all go to? That's what we were always asking ourselves! And I still don't know. It did cost John a lot to commute and go to work, to keep up appearances, I guess. A Mercedes, lunches, good clothes—but I could never understand how he'd take a hundred dollars one day for pocket money, and two days later he didn't know where it went to. This is what we'd argue about. His pocket money. Never left us without, but he'd just keep cashing checks, and once in a while I would look at the checking account and I didn't know where the hell it was all going to."

John interrupted me, saying, "It was in a good cause."

"If I spend fifty dollars, I can just about account for every one of those dollars. Even if it's over a period of a month, I know where that fifty went to. But he could never do that. That was our biggest problem. He'd say to me, 'You must have sent me to the store.' Or 'I must've bought a bottle of Scotch or something.' And then he'd search for the money! Look all over the house for it. Then come to me and say, 'Ah, forget about it, Ann. I must've put gas in the car.' That was his biggest out. Gas money!"

*JOHN*   I had to keep restraining myself from interrupting, so I was glad when Sylvia turned back to me and asked me about my job.

"Did you feel secure? Or did you dread working there? Do you think the pressure of your job contributed to your coronary?"

"I understand why you're asking these questions. Let me just say that I was *very* secure there. As a matter of fact, if I hadn't had my heart attack, I would have been my boss's replacement. No doubt about it. See, it was set up in such a way that you had to designate who your replacement was going to be—in the event that you were going to leave, or be transferred. So you had to be constantly training the person who you thought was capable of replacing you. Because it was such a rapidly expanding company —you could be here one day and transferred the next. I always felt secure in my job. And felt secure that if my boss were to leave, that I would have his job."

"It didn't worry you that if you were ever to be fired, they'd have your replacement right at hand?"

"I never gave it a second thought. Unless there was some politics involved."

"Was there any politics involved?"

"No. And as far as any job pressures contributing to my coronary, I would have to say no. If stress were to bring on a heart attack, it should have happened in Puerto Rico when they first sent me down there, in the early sixties. I was working fourteen, sixteen hours a day, seven days a week, for a solid straight year, working alongside the Puerto Ricans. I don't think the pressures of the job *in any way* brought the attack on. Or hastened it. I really don't. Because I've always been the type of a person that had a lot of drive. I've worked hard my whole life."

*ANN* When Sylvia turned to me and asked if I thought John's job had anything to do with his heart condition, I had to disagree with John.

"Pressure. Work. Home. Support a family. Demands. I don't know about his bosses because I know he got along so well with them, but I know the pressures at work were to keep ahead and on your toes so nobody steps on *you*—or steps over you. And the pressure of the cost of living, to pay the bills for the things that you like or the things that you need, to keep up with the Joneses. I never felt that way. But John. That's another story. He likes to keep up. According to our means, or above them."

John looked at me like he was annoyed. "What's wrong with that?"

"But I do want to say something important here, Sylvia. And that is, that he's done it all by himself. He only has two years of college. He's really worked hard. It wasn't who you knew. It was really the work he did. He would never climb over anybody to get ahead. But he wouldn't knuckle under to anybody, either. Whatever he did, he did straight out. Right up front. Nothing under the table. No favors for a favor. And we knew that kind of thing went on a lot. But John is his own man."

"I understand." She wrote something down. "And now that he's retired, what kind of adjustment has John made?"

I had to think about that for a few seconds.

"Did you ever meet somebody who's been in the military

service and keeps rehashing stories about it? *This* is John. He keeps reminiscing about work. He loves the job. I really think that now that he's not working, it's hard on him. He keeps in touch constantly with his old boss and pal, Jim Clark. Jim's like a brother to John. Keeps him up to date on everything that goes on at Sea-Land. All of Sea-Land. All the divisions. And they still treat him like an employee. Send him brochures, and he reads them from cover to cover. But he's never gone back to company headquarters. I think it's because he can't face his former associates. He's *very* competitive. John's a very competitive person."

"Getting back to you, Ann, how do you bear up under the strain? It can't be easy."

"No, it isn't."

"Do you ever wonder if somehow *you're* being punished for something *you* might have done?"

"Lately I've been wondering . . . why I've been punished . . . or my children were being punished. What did I ever do in life? I always felt I never did any harm to anybody else. Never. And I still question it. But I do believe there is a God. For a while there I have to admit I doubted it, when John was so sick. But I do believe. Otherwise, John wouldn't still be here. There *has* to be a God."

**JOHN** The next time we talked, we were in my room. I had some free time between tests, and no other patients were in the room with us. Sylvia pulled over a chair and sat down. She was carrying a notebook and pen. Ann was sitting on the bed next to me. And the first question she asked us took us a little bit by surprise.

"John, Ann, do you have any *regrets*?"

Ann looked at her like maybe she wasn't real. "What a question!"

I didn't see any irony in her question, though. I said, "Maybe . . . in a way. I envy a young couple—who has just gotten married, and haven't had any children for maybe the first ten years of their married life, and have the freedom to go wherever they want to, every weekend, to go away. I could say that I could look back and I might be envious of them. Because we don't have the freedom to do that. Janice was conceived two years after we were married. We were gonna wait five years. But after we got married, we pushed it up a little. Looking back now, it was probably because all our friends were having children. It was maybe the 'in' thing to do. To have children."

Later in the week, we had a discussion in the conference room. Again, it was Sylvia, Ann, and me. This time Sylvia went for the brass ring.

"John . . . do you have a drinking problem? Are you an alcoholic?"

I looked at both of them for a moment. "I don't consider myself an alcoholic. I find a drink very relaxing to me. Even when I was working, I'd come home at night and I'd sit down and have a drink or two before dinner. At work I'd maybe have a few drinks at lunch. But not every day. Of course it would depend on where you went for lunch. Sometimes you went to a place that didn't serve liquor. If they served drinks, we'd have a few before our lunch. But we were going to that restaurant because we enjoyed their *food. Not for their drinks.*

"I don't feel that I *have* to have a drink. I enjoy a drink. And if I'm gonna have a drink, I enjoy a strong drink. I'd get home from work maybe eight o'clock at night. Frankly, I'm confused by some of these things you see on television asking, 'Are you an alcoholic?' I think Ann has a hangup about it."

Whereupon Ann retaliated, by saying something like, "John, you're an alcoholic if you can't get through the day without a drink. You're an alcoholic if you have to have a drink before you face any pressures. You're an alcoholic if you have to have a drink before you have company. Or if you're going to a party."

I said, "Ahem. Point of order, here. Equal time for the defense, please. The party that she's referring to was next door. It was a younger, more different group than we're used to. Not hippies or anything. More Mod. They don't have the same philosophy or thinking that I have. They're a lot more liberal about sex, clothing, even bigotry. I've always been brought up with respect for law and order, authority, the elderly. And I don't agree, for instance, that cops are pigs. That night, those people and I just didn't have that much in common. One was a lawyer. One was a commercial artist. One is a contractor. But their attitudes didn't make me angry. As a matter of fact, I got *smashed*! I don't feel any better than those people. I don't look down at 'em or up at 'em or anything else. It's just that I don't feel we have anything in common, say, to sit down and shoot the breeze. I could sit down with someone and talk all night long without having a drink."

"I don't believe that remark, John darling."

At that point I called Ann a traitor, because she said she didn't honestly believe I would sit down all night with *anybody* without a drink.

"Unless it was with the planning board," she said. "I know most everybody we know is the same way. You go to somebody's house, it's, 'How about a drink?' I used to offer coffee. I don't even *bother* to offer coffee any more, unless their wives are with them. No one wants coffee. 'Would you like a drink?' 'Yes! What've you got?' But John doesn't drink as much any more. He could go to a party and in a matter of three hours put away a *quart* of Scotch."

Then I said, "Every New Year's Eve we'd never leave the lake. We'd have the clubhouse up there, and I've always felt, why go out and expose yourself on the highway to the rest of the drunks on the road? You bring your own bottle. And if it's a dinner, they supply the dinner and the food. I *have* drunk in excess of twenty martinis in one night. And still known what I'm doing. And not be laying on the floor. After you have three or four, it doesn't matter any more. You feel relaxed. More open. More candid. You get a glow on. It was the driving that bothered Ann, though. It always has."

She told Sylvia, I'd had three totals. And walked away from every one of them. Which was true. But I said, "I haven't had one in a long time now.

"I had an accident one night, when I was driving. After I had quite a few to drink. And how the hell I ever got on this road where this accident occurred I still don't know to this day! It's nowhere on the route home! I must've taken a wrong turn or something. I didn't know where the hell I was!"

Ann was getting upset. She said, "See? He's making a joke out of it. The police called me. And I called my brother-in-law, to go get him. Three o'clock in the morning. 'Go get John.' Then I realized that I'd forgotten which *town* they told me he was at. So I had to call four different police barracks to find out where he was! Finally I spoke to the Netcong state troopers, and they told me he was down in Liberty Corners."

"Like I say, I was drinking. And I ran off the road. And I tore maybe ten mailboxes down in a row. This is when I had the Mercedes, thank God. It was a good solid car. And I ended up on the other side of this small narrow road. The lights go on, and all the neighbors come running out in their pajamas and robes, to see what in the hell all the racket is about. And then the cops came and they had me walking up and down the painted line in the highway to see if I could walk straight. They were trying to prove I was drunk. I told 'em I'd gotten a blowout! One tire was gone because I'd hit this big boulder. That's what *stopped* me! So this cop has me out in the middle of the road walking up and down the center line. Then he has me bringing my right hand up to my nose, and my left hand to my nose, and there's a big crowd standing around me pointing to their smashed mailboxes. You feel like a fool! Needless to say, I sobered up pretty fast. He gave me a ticket for crossing the center line."

"Were there any other incidents like this?"

"No. I'm pretty careful."

"But John only flies when he drinks. Not half smashed. He's got to be *completely* smashed!"

"Listen, I've had some flights! I come up from Puerto Rico one time, I was on a night flight, first time I ever took a night flight, and a lot of PR's that come up to New York are on those flights. They *crate* them in there! And they have their chickens and everything else with them, and all of a sudden the engines start coughing—and at the same time we're just *diving, straight down*! And I think, Oh Lord, this is it! Oh . . . Jeez! This is *IT*! Now, I've been in air pockets before, but I never saw *anything* like this, or ever heard such an ungodly noise before, from the motors—plus we just kept falling for I don't know how many thousands of feet. We went down, down, down, and down. And *finally* you could hear the engines snap in. Well, I was sitting next to two PR's, and the two of them are *STONED*. They each had a fifth of rum with them, and when that happened I literally *grabbed* the bottle away from one of them and hoisted it—*STRAIGHT UP*! Well, they're very emotional people, and there was *PANIC* on that plane. The people and the chickens are just screaming and carrying on like some kind of *friggin' barnyard*! *Terrible*!"

Then Sylvia says, "John, this is one of those damned-if-you-do, and damned-if-you-don't questions."

"That seems to be your specialty."

"How do you feel about Ann? What could you tell me?"

"How do I feel about Ann? I don't even have to think about

that. Ann's gone through more than I have. She's put up with more. I really mean that. She's suffered more, emotionally. You couldn't believe it. You couldn't ask for a more dedicated person. I don't know *anybody* that would put up with what she's had to put up with. She's never left my side. We have an expression between us, that says it all: *It would take ten niggers to replace her!*"

We all laughed.

Then she asked Ann how she would describe me. "How would you describe him, if I'd never met him before?"

Ann says, "Hmmmmmmmm. *That's* a trick question! Well, I'd say that John is tall, medium in build, with dark hair. He's got green eyes. And he's extremely good looking. Extremely. There's no flies on John. Weighs about two hundred pounds. Likes to dress well, conservatively. Never a hair out of place. Also, he smiles a lot. Watch out for that smile!"

My turn next. Sylvia says, "John? Can you describe Ann for me? And your children?"

"Ann is five feet eight inches tall, has brown eyes, weighs one hundred twenty pounds, and is very attractive. She has brown eyes and brown hair, frosted with reddish highlights. She wouldn't know that I notice these things. She likes nice stylish clothes.

Our oldest is Janice. She's sixteen. She's very slender. Very quiet. She's a very good student. Our little Joanie is six years old. Terror on wheels. She's very mischievous. But she's extremely generous. Loves her tap and ballet lessons. John Junior is seventeen months younger, weighs all of forty pounds, is very tall for his age, has a shock of blond hair, a great smile, and is very good looking. He'll be King of the Drive-ins some day."

"Just like his old man," said Ann.

"He was born on Saint Patrick's Day."

"From the day I conceived, he called it. 'You wouldn't dare

have a child of mine in March, and not have it on Saint Patrick's Day!' In fact, when I woke up with back pain, and I felt the baby moving around, I said to myself, 'It can't be! It's Saint Patrick's Day! I'll be goddammed! The bastard called it!' "

"And one month after little John was born, I had my heart attack. So you can see it was quite shocking! Ann wanted to name him John Edward Hurley, after me. But I said, 'No, sir. It's going to be John *Patrick* Hurley!' And that's what we named him. And he's a beautiful boy."

# 13

## Yes

*JOHN*  On Friday, November 15th, they gave me the final tests. And after the last blood workup, Dr. Schroeder and a small group of doctors, four of them, took me into a tiny conference room. They asked me questions such as, "Why do you want to become a transplant?" "What are your specific reasons?" I told them basically that it was because of my family situation, that I had small children, and I wanted the transplant to prolong my life as long as possible.

They took everything in. They'd ask more questions, but wouldn't respond with anything in return. I had the feeling that they had already made up their minds about me but were just proceeding according to the rules and carrying out certain formalities.

After about thirty minutes of this, they brought me down to the ward, and I got into my bed. Ann was there. Dr. Schroeder pulled the curtain around my bed and suddenly became very serious.

"John, Ann. You've been accepted as a recipient for a heart transplant."

I felt relieved and anxious at the same time.

"The alternative to surgery is this: If you don't elect to have the transplant, our test results indicate that you have anywhere from two weeks to six months . . . on the outside . . . to live. The damage to your heart is severe. However the rest of your organs are in excellent shape. In top shape. The operation itself is relatively simple, believe it or not. By using two groups of surgeons, working simultaneously, we just remove the normal heart from the donor. At the same time, your circulation is taken over by a heart-lung machine, and your damaged heart is removed from you, by opening up the pericardial sac, and severing all the veins and arteries holding it in place. The whole heart is removed, with its four chambers, four valves, the stumps of the two main arteries, and its self-contained nerve system. Then we sew the new heart into place in your body. An electric shock gets it going again, and that's it."

Then Dr. Schroeder put his hand on my shoulder for a second.

"John, you must understand, we're not offering you immortality. At best, we're offering you the *possibility* of living longer than you normally would be expected to, under the present circumstances. There is a one-third chance of your not getting off the operating table at all. There is a one-third chance of getting off the table with some sort of physical damage, like a stroke, or brain damage. I won't minimize the risks for you. And there's a one-third chance of your getting off the table with everything being perfectly OK."

"I see."

"And the medications that we would be giving you, to manage and prevent a rejection of the new heart . . . those medications themselves often have severe side effects. Again, we won't minimize the risks for you."

"I appreciate that. And I understand."

"Then, if you get off the table OK, the chances are in your favor that everything will be all right for the first seventy-two hours. After seventy-two hours, there is the possibility of *anything* happening, such as an infection setting in, or a total rejection. This is the time of the greatest risk. You have a one-third chance of making it to six months. If you live for the first six months, the odds increase to fifty percent in your favor that you'll live for the next six months. After one year the odds decrease to forty percent that you'll survive for another year. After the second year, it's thirty percent in your favor. And so on, up until five years, which is the basis for our current statistical information. Of course, there are exceptions, people who have lived longer than five years."

"Pretty grim, isn't it?"

"John, you're dying. We'd like to do something for you. We'd like you and Ann to give this all some serious thought, and let us know if you want us to go ahead. Unless you have any further questions?"

"No. Not really. You say those drugs have serious side effects?"

"For preventive immunosuppression. Yes. They do. Among other things, they can cause osteoporosis, hepatotoxicity, and bone marrow depression leading to thrombocytopenia and leukopenia. And all of the other side effects associated with long-term steroid therapy."

"Oh. Great. Not a very thrilling choice."

"No indeed. There are risks. No doubt about that. You've got to choose among the alternatives."

They all walked out the door. I looked at Ann. She looked at me. We shook our heads at the same time.

"Whew! Some great choice I have!"

"But it's a chance, isn't it?"

"I guess it is. It's the only one I've got."

We thought for a few minutes. We knew what we were going to say. There really was no other choice. A chance for life is a *chance*. No matter what the risks. Where there's life, there's hope. And believe me, when you're in this position, you grab for it. For any kind of a lifeline. You reach out and grab for it. With *both fists*.

Ann went out into the hallway, and in a moment Dr. Schroeder returned with her.

"Our answer is yes, Doc."

"All right, John. We'll go ahead with it. We don't have any donors on hand at present, so tomorrow morning we'll discharge you, and you'll stay at the motel . . . or let us know where you're going to be, and we'll be in contact with you if and when a donor becomes available."

We shook hands, and he left. Ann took my hand and held on to it for a good long time.

That evening, Ann left the hospital, planning to come back the next morning with my clothes, to check me out. But no sooner had she left, when in comes a nurse—it was 10:00 p.m.—and she says, "Mr. Hurley, I think you'd better call your wife. Because they've changed their minds. They're not going to discharge you tomorrow morning."

I look at her, my heart pounding. "Why not?"

"Because . . . there's a possibility . . . that we have a donor available for you. A new heart."

I was just completely stunned. "You're not serious!"

"It's just a possibility. But they don't want to discharge you, in case they're going to have to operate."

I sat there in shock. My mouth got so dry I could hardly swallow. After I had gone through that hell week, I was really looking forward to spending at least *some* time out in a motel with Ann, alone. Now it was like someone had just pronounced the death sentence.

I had been in bed watching television. Next to me was this fire chief who was in there for a suspected heart attack. So this nurse says, "You'd better call your wife now and let her know. Or do you want *me* to call her?"

I just sat there . . . and finally said, "No. There's no sense in calling her. She's probably just getting ready for bed. If I tell her now, she's not gonna sleep all night long. And if they do the transplant tomorrow, it's gonna be rough enough on her. She's gonna be up and not sleeping anyway."

So I didn't call. I just sat there, *numb*.

The nurse says, "They've scheduled it so that they'll be flying up the donor's body by helicopter. It's due to arrive at six in the morning. Then they'll do the workup, matching his tissues to yours. And if everything matches, and it's a suitable heart, the operation will be performed tomorrow."

I didn't sleep that night at all.

This fire chief that was in the next bed, he sort of kept me company—all night long—talking and trying to get my mind off it. We were smoking. His wife was keeping him well supplied. I think I smoked a whole pack that night. I told him, "I'm a little nervous about this whole thing." He says to me, "If I were you, I *know* I'd be feeling mighty nervous about it, too."

So we talked about anything and everything that night. His job. My job. He was the fire chief at Stanford University. They have a tremendous campus and have to have their own fire department. He had been in the Navy too. So we talked about where he was stationed, the different bases, what ships we were on. Like that. He did a good job of trying to take my mind off things. It's funny, what things come back to you at a time like that. The memories.

I remembered I got my first car when I was in the Navy. This was 1954 to 1956. It was a '51 Mercury V-8. With Mercomatic transmission. A great car. I only wish I could get my hands on one now. Jet black. Had a finish on it like a Cadillac limousine. Highly lacquered paint. It was a beauty. I was always working on it, shining it up, over and over, with a chamois cloth and Simoniz. A classic. A real heavy car. I could take that thing out on the Belt Parkway and go 120 miles an hour with no trouble at all, just holding the road.

While I was stationed in Virginia, I used to drive back and forth to New York. It took twelve hours driving. In order to pay for gas and tolls, I'd pick up a load of sailors at the bus station on Forty-second Street, and charge them five bucks a head. The bus fare was fourteen dollars, so they were saving money.

We were stationed at the Naval Base in Norfolk, home of the Amphibs. I'd get off Friday afternoon, at 4:00, on a 72-hour pass. By the time I got home and drove over to the local gin mill and had a couple of beers with my buddies, and bullshit with them, I'd just *maybe* get to bed that night. And maybe I wouldn't. And pretty soon, that whole weekend would be up. Come Sunday night, I'd leave at 4:00 p.m. and head back to Virginia. I also used to hitchhike quite a bit those weeks when I didn't have enough money for gas. Which of course took a lot longer, because you never knew *when* you'd be getting home. So I used to give blood.

It was Navy procedure that if you gave blood on Friday morning, you were then allowed to leave at noon, instead of at 4:00. So whatever opportunity that we had to give blood—it could be every eight weeks—I'd give my pint of blood. Then we'd drink our orange juice, eat our doughnut (which was standard fare at ceremonies like this), pick up our pay, and run like hell out to the highway to start hitchhiking home.

Well, this one time I left the base at noon, and come *midnight,* I'm still only in Maryland! And these two chippies pick me up.

And they were older. Maybe mid-twenties. They drive by and they're coming from a dance. And they're stoned. One was a big fat babe, with mangy dark hair. The other was a good-looking blonde with a great mouth.

When they first stopped the car, they asked me: "Hey sailor! Where are you going?" I told 'em, "I'm going to Brooklyn!" So they say, "Hop in. We'll give you a ride."

This was on Route 13. And all of a sudden the car veers off onto a side road, and we start driving down a series of narrow back roads. The first thing that goes through my mind was a fear of getting mugged. I'd heard about that kind of thing being pretty common. And I'd just been paid. And I'm saying, "Hey listen. Where are you going? I'm going to Brooklyn. Better let me out here." And fatty says, "Don't worry about it. We'll take you back to the highway. Don't worry."

So they take me up to this private house. Fatty's house. And they say, "C'mon in. We'll have some coffee or something." Turns out they were out of coffee. So we had a drink. And the next thing I know, I'm upstairs.

As to who got whose clothes off first, it was probably a tie. Actually, the good-looking one was first. We jumped into bed and she was as quick as a bunny. I didn't have to do a thing but lie back and enjoy. It was like Mercomatic transmission!

An hour later, she left. I never got her name. And then I was left alone with fatty. She owned the house. I wanted to get out of there right then, but I didn't know where the hell I was, or which direction to hitch. I figured she'd be driving me out to the highway later, so I stayed. She climbs into bed with me, and boy was she big. Like a whale. And boy did she stink! She'd been dancing all night and had worked up a sweat. But she made it interesting, anyway. I'll give her that.

Must have been five in the morning—I hear the milkman

puttering around downstairs. So I creep out of bed, slide on my uniform, tiptoe downstairs, and whispering, so fatty won't hear me upstairs, I *beg* him to give me a ride out to the main highway. He takes one look at me, standing there in the moonlight, without my shoes on, not even zipped up yet, looking like an escapee from a nut house, and it's a wonder he didn't run away from me! I guess he realized I was harmless, so he obliged.

Maybe it was the uniform?

Next I went on the communications ship *Adirondack*. It was a flagship for the Amphibs. I was a gunner's mate. The majority of the time we were attached to the Caribbean area. I spent a lot of time in Puerto Rico, Cuba, and St. Thomas. You know the picture *Away All Boats*? Jeff Chandler starred in it. We participated in the filming. Our ship and crew. They shot it off St. Thomas. I met Jeff Chandler. He came into this one bar down there, the Delilah Bar, and bought drinks for a bunch of us. Stayed all night long, kibitzing, picking up the tab for everyone. Hell of a nice guy. Sang "Blue Moon" in that great baritone of his, solo.

After that, I had shore duty. Became an instructor at Little Creek, Virginia, on the LCVPs. These are landing crafts, the boats that take the Marines onto the beachheads, and the front drops down and the gung-ho Marines storm onto shore. My job was to instruct those Marines in how to drive the boats, get over sandbars, dock them, land them along the beach, and drop the ramp down. We used to have some good times.

I remember we'd take these Marines out for practice—at midnight—in the dead of winter. Freezing our tusheys off! Gung-ho Marines, right? No moon out, and you couldn't see a thing. And for some reason they always picked the coldest goddamn night you could possibly have. Now, we knew, from making all the landings, where all the sandbars were. So what we used to do is —we'd hit the first sandbar, gun the engines to get over it, then proceed in to the beachhead. Then, once you get in to the beachhead, you'd drop the ramp, and all these Marines would go screaming out of the boat and onto the beach. This was part of their war games. I think they were also screaming about how cold it was.

So what we used to do, once in a while, was—we'd hit the first sandbar and *pretend* we were already at the beach! And drop the ramp! And these guys were in full battle dress! And they'd go *charging*—right up to their necks—into the ocean! Then we'd back the boat up real fast, and get the hell outta there! They'd be yelling after us: "FUCK YOU, YOU DIRTY COCKSUCKERS! COME BACK HERE YOU MUTHAFUCKING DOUCHEBAGS! WE'LL GET YOUR ASSES FOR THIS, YOU DIRTY ROTTEN BASTARDS!"

Another time, we were attached to shore duty, putting the ship out of commission, and we were living on a house barge, which is a barracks on water, standing three stories high. And this friend of mine, Weinstein, and I went out, went into the local PX, and got all slopped up. I mean *stoned.*

Al Weinstein was a good buddy of mine. The only Jew I ever knew who wanted to become a professional boxer. He was a middleweight. And we went all over the world together. Well, Al and me, we come back to the ship (and this is like two in the morning). And we're stumbling around on the top deck, trying to find our room. We couldn't even find our *key,* let alone our room! And there were these deck chairs that kept getting in our way. The most annoying damn thing. Everywhere you walked, you'd be bumping into one of them. Well, I hit one of them, right across my shinbone, and saw stars it hurt so much. I got so pissed off at this, I just picked up the chair and threw it over the side into the river! Then Weinstein, he's so pissed off that *I'm* pissed off, *he* picks up a chair and throws it after the first one! Well, we ended up throwing *ten chairs* over! Then we threw *six fire extinguishers* over! Then we started throwing guys' *sea-bags* with all their *clothes* over! And everybody's living out of those sea-bags, since we had no lockers!

Then we went to bed and passed out.

Unbeknownst to us, the river was patrolled, constantly. And they see these bags come floating down the river, and naturally they assumed that a boat had capsized, and some sailors had drowned. So they got the sea-bags and traced them to the barge. And the next thing we know, these MPs are waking Weinstein and me up. They knew just who to talk to. The two wise-asses.

"You guys are really gonna get your asses hung now!"

And I said "Whattaya mean? What did *we* do?"

But we were the last guys to come back on board ship, and they had us nailed. They gave us a Summary Court Martial. And this wasn't funny at all. During the trial, they asked me if I had anything to say. I said, "I'm just standing mute, Sir. I have no defense. And no excuse."

"And what about you, Weinstein?"

"Same thing, Sir. No defense. No excuse."

We got three months' hard labor. But fortunately, hard labor wasn't like Leavenworth. They just had us doing the shit details. Putting the ship out of commission, like cleaning the shit out of the bilges. And we were restricted, so we couldn't leave the ship.

But besides the hard labor, and not leaving the ship, the guys whose sea-bags were involved were ready to *kill us*! We had to have all of their clothes dry-cleaned. And pay back over a thousand dollars in property costs.

But I really liked the Navy. Once, in the Far East, Weinstein tells me about this place in Taiwan, up in the mountains, some cabbie had told him about. "John, so help me they give you these *baths*—in the natural springs that they got up there. We got to go!" So we went. At first I was scared. When I was a kid, I used to think that the sexiest women in the whole world were the Oriental girls. I probably got this from the movies. And the Dragon Lady, from "Terry and the Pirates."

So Weinstein and I, we go into this Oriental type of a medium-sized palace, and we don't know what to expect. Weinstein looks around at the huge rooms we're going through, and there seems to be actual gold running through the paint on the walls, glass, and ceilings. And candles burning everywhere.

He says to me as we're being guided by this old lady who looks like a high priestess of some sort: "Jeez, John! Would you look at this joint?"

All I can think of to say is, "Holy cow!"

The high priestess shows us into this undressing area and holds out her hand. "Ten dollar please."

We go through our pockets and fish out five apiece. We hand the bills to her. She takes them, examines them, and nods negatively. "Ten dollar *EACH*."

We fork over another couple of bills. Then she motions for us to go behind this curtain to get undressed, and she hands us these white robes to put on afterwards. We finish in one minute flat. We're anxious by now.

So we step out, wearing these robes, and I'm feeling like I'm wearing somebody's borrowed nightie, and the high priestess beckons us to follow her. We walk down this series of steps and past a lot of tall pillars and archways. And we can feel the temperature getting much warmer. Like you were entering a steam room, or sauna. Then she motions for us to enter this chamber room, where you can see steam coming from. I look at Weinstein, and in we go.

We walk down about ten or fifteen steps, and there are the girls. Two for each of us. And we couldn't believe what we saw. What a bunch of *dogs*! Unbelievable! They looked like Sumo wrestlers! Weinstein looks at me and his jaw drops in amazement. "I want my money back!"

They had shorts on, and T-shirts, and except for the breasts and the slanty eyes, they looked exactly like the guys we'd been saluting on board ship all year long! They certainly weren't your geisha types. But before we could say another word, they took charge. And tended strictly to business. They took us out of our robes, and there was no hanky-panky whatsoever.

One of my girls says to me, "Special minerals in water. Straighten you out real good." Weinstein hears this and says, "I certainly hope so." Then she says, "Ancient Oriental cleansing rituals make you in natural harmony with nature again." They washed us down, with soap and sponges, and Weinstein is giving me the winks. Then they moved us to long flat wooden tables, to give us a massage.

Weinstein says, "Ah hah! Here it comes. Watch out."

But it didn't. It was the real thing. Just designed to make our muscles relax all over. Without any sex involvement. Weinstein looked surprised. Then pleased.

They hauled us off the tables and washed us down again. Only this time it was with ice water! We started jumping up and down, shivering, like we were at the North Pole. Weinstein says to me, "These people are sadists! Are you sure they're the *Allies*? I gotta get the hell outta here! This is *freezing ridiculous*!"

Then the girls led us to the final rinse area. They poured large wooden buckets of warm water all over us, till the steam was rising around us. Then they toweled us down from top to bottom, using very strong, vigorous motions and really getting the blood going. It was invigorating! I swear you could go in there *stoned,* come out of there *sober,* go to bed, sleep for three hours, and get up and feel like a million bucks! That's how great those girls and their rituals were.

# 14

## And Counting

*JOHN* The fire chief heard the helicopter first. He tapped me on the hand, and I heard it too, coming closer and closer in for a landing.

You'd be surprised how fast that night went. The fire chief and I had stayed up that whole night, just talking. I still had this picture of Weinstein in my mind when I realized once again that I was in my hospital room, waiting for—what?

I felt very nervous.

The TV was still on, without the sound, playing some kind of Charlie Chan movie. And for a second, I really missed Weinstein. I had lost track of him after we got out of service and haven't seen or heard from him since. We were good buddies. He would have had something funny to say now, to brighten things up for me.

I looked at my watch. It was 6:30 a.m. Saturday, November 16th. I could hear that chopper coming closer and closer to the landing pad now, and my heart quickened. I knew that the donor was definitely being brought in. It touched down, you could hear it nearby, and I knew the countdown had begun. Now it would just be a matter of time before they knew if they would operate on me or not.

I called Ann.

*ANN*  The phone rang. I jumped up out of bed. I had been sound asleep. I heard his voice.

"What's the matter, John? Did anything go wrong?"

And he says, "Ann. Look. Don't bring my clothes."

And I said, "Why?" I took a look outside. It was still dark out.

"Nothing's wrong. I'm just not going to be released from the hospital yet."

"Why? What's wrong? What happened?"

And he said, "Well . . . they might have a donor."

And I said, "You're kidding! Come on, John. You're kidding!"

"I'm not kidding. I'm serious. They've already brought him in, on a helicopter."

I said, "John, if you're kidding me, I'll kill you! You got me outta bed to tell me *that*?" Those were my exact words.

He says, "I'm not kidding, Ann. Don't get upset. Just c'mon over. Be here with me."

And I said, "OK."

I hung up the phone, went into the bathroom, and started washing my hair. It didn't need washing. I'd had it done at the beauty parlor the day before. And suddenly I realized what I was doing. My God, I'm washing my hair! What am I doing? I've got to get to the hospital and I'm washing my hair!

I started drying my hair and trying to get dressed in a hurry, and the phone rings again. It was John.

"Hello. Ann?"

And I said, "You son-of-a-bitch! You *were* kidding me!"

"No, no, no. I'm not kidding. I just called to tell you not to call anybody at home. Because it's only a *possible* donor. It can't be definite until they do all their tests."

So I said, "All right, I'll be right over."

I got to the hospital in less than half an hour. And when I got there, it was still only a possibility. So I called Jackie and Mike Ladner right away. They came down within an hour. The three of us sat in the waiting room all day, waiting. We talked about our Caribbean cruise to the islands, the year before. Jackie had brought her scrapbook of vacation pictures down in an album, and we went over the pictures.

Rehashing everything was the best thing for us. Although John had been so sick, he never let on to anybody, and put on a good enough front so that we did have a few good moments. One picture brought it back.

We had been in Curacao, at the Hilton. The pool there was shaped like the Star of David. And it was so cold that day, so freezing cold, that all John and Mike did was wade into the pool —and *piss* in it! With their backs to us. It was so cold, they were the only ones in the pool. And Jackie snapped a picture of them while they were doing it.

Another picture, taken on the *Carla "C"* touring the islands. Jackie was swimming on board ship, and there was a slide. John had dared her to go down the slide. So she did. And when she hit the water, the top of her bathing suit flew off! Well, she's really stacked. And everybody around the pool just cracked up laughing, and started applauding. John yelled out, "Encore! Encore! Encore!" Jackie just readjusted herself after she found the top, and went right on swimming. We had a picture of that, too.

By this time Jackie and I were giggling hysterically. Finally Mike got exasperated with us.

"This is no way to act in a hospital! Do you realize the tremendous pressure on John? And the two of you are sitting here laughing and joking like a couple of hyenas!"

I turned to him and said, "Look, Mike. I don't know what to say. I think it's good for us to try to laugh. What should we do? Sit here and cry?"

Then a nurse came over to us. "Mrs. Hurley?"

"Yes?"

"It's definite. Your husband is going to be operated on. This afternoon."

I went to a pay phone, called home, and spoke to my sister Barbara. Then I called my sister-in-law Joan in Florida.

Then Dr. Schroeder comes over. "Mrs. Hurley. Uh . . . there's been a delay. The operation may not be performed today after all. There's one test that must be repeated. Certain things are not matching up, and we have to repeat the test by taking more blood samples from John."

A few minutes later, Joan calls back and wants to know what time the operation has been scheduled for.

"Joan, you won't believe this, but just this second it's all been canceled again."

"What do you mean canceled?" She got all upset and started to cry. "What are you trying to do to me? Make me crazy?"

"Joan, please. They told us it was all set to go, and now they tell me it isn't. They have to run some more tests. Only when they're sure are they gonna operate on him."

"I'm coming anyway. I'll be on the first flight I can get."

And while she was still on the phone with me, Dr. Schroeder came back in and touched me on the shoulder. "Mrs. Hurley?"

"Just a minute, Joan. Hold on a second."

"Mrs. Hurley, the surgery is scheduled for three o'clock. The tests worked out fine. And everything is Go."

*JOHN* My room became very solemn.

All the other patients were looking over at me pretty often. Nobody had said anything about it. But the word had spread. When Ann got there, with Jackie and Mike, they all just stared at her, then quickly over to me. Nobody spoke for a while, there was so much tension in the room. And when they finally were able, it was all small talk. "Hello. How are you?" And shut right up. No conversations. The other patients just whispered among themselves. I think they were all very nervous and afraid to upset me in any way. They didn't want to intrude.

The nurses wouldn't give me anything to eat at all. Just a cup of coffee and a piece of toast.

Then in comes this British doctor who's in charge of the cell-matching team, and with him is my friend, the gypsy girl technician who pierced my ear earlier in the week. Still wearing her turban, rather than a nurse's hat. She comes in, and I'm not kidding and I'm not exaggerating—she's got two tubes with needles on the end that must be *eight* inches long! And I say to her, "And what are you gonna do with *those*?"

And she says, "We need to take some blood."

"Some blood? All week they've been taking blood outta me! An hour ago they were just in here and took out *six* tubes of blood! Now *you* need some blood? Come on! Let's be *reasonable* about this, can't we? How about leaving a little for *me*?"

"This is the most important part. To find out if the match is there."

"So what have you people been doing with this stuff before now? Flushing it down the toilet?"

So I watch her suck these two gigantic needles full of blood out of me. Didn't hurt me. Just *worried* me. Then she's got these flasks, or beakers, whatever you call them—the kind you put on Bunsen burners in high school—and each one must hold a pint. And she pours the tubes of blood right there in front of me, into the flasks. There are these beads of something in each flask. And she puts a cork in each one of these things, and she's standing over me with these beakers, and she's shaking and shaking the blood back and forth and back and forth—and I swear, man, this is *VOODOO*! You know, here's this girl with a turban on, standing there with these two beakers going and my blood is inside them going around in there like a chocolate malted!

I look up at the doctor, who is supervising this extravaganza, and I say to him, "What the hell do you people do with all the excess?"

He didn't smile. And no sooner do I say this when in comes *another* nurse, and she's gonna take *more* blood! And she's got *fourteen* test tubes with her! *Jeezus!* At first I'm not saying a word. She comes in, carrying a little case, and she starts laying out these test tubes, in rows, on the bed. She looks at me for a second, then looks away. I give her the gimlet eye.

"Aw *c'mon*! What are you guys *trying to do to me*?"

And she says "Oh. Nothing. We're just gonna take a little blood."

I turn to her, count the test tubes one by one, then look her straight in the eye. She looks away. Then I look up at the doctor, and then at the gypsy, and I make my announcement.

"Baby, I don't give a damn *what* happens, you ain't getting one goddamn more ounce of blood outta me! You can call anyone you want. You can tell them the patient is *tapped* out. The blood bank is closed! Finito! Done! Finished! Kaput! There is no more blood going outta me. Case *closed*!"

After she finished filling up the fourteenth test tube, the orderly came in to prep me. He must have been 6'7" tall, a big black fellow. Very thin. "Hi. My name is Robert." He pulls the curtains around the bed and proceeds to shave all the hair off my body. Lathers me all down with Phisohex soap, and uses a safety razor. From my neck to my mid-thigh, I looked like a plucked chicken.

Then old Sergeant Nurse comes in to inspect. She parts the curtains and looks me up and down. I look at her. "Can't you *knock*?" She winks at me and says, "Listen Hurley, what you've got I've seen before." Then she tells Robert, "That isn't enough. Lower. Shave him lower." Robert looks at her and says, "They're not operating on his *knees.*" Sarge sneers at him and says, "Lower."

So he shaves me lower. To below my knees. And when he finished, Ann, Jackie, and Mike came back into the room, and Jackie says, "How far did they shave you, pal?"

"From my neck to my knees."

"And what kinda transplant you say they're gonna do on you, John?"

A nurse comes in and hands me a release form to sign. It's to donate my organs. In case anything goes wrong. I had told them, "If this thing doesn't work out, I want all my vital organs donated. And my corneas."

After I finished signing it, she thanked me and told me, "You'll be going upstairs soon, Mr. Hurley."

"How do you mean that, nurse?"

She turned red. "Oh, not the way you think."

"I certainly hope not."

At that point I'm on forty milligrams of Valium. But when they tell me I'm gonna go up for the operation, I say, "Gimme something to quiet me down." So Sergeant Nurse, she gives me a five-milligram tablet of Valium!

"Lady, you're joking! All along I've been taking *forty* milligrams a day to keep me quiet, and now you're gonna give me *five*—to calm me down before my heart gets *transplanted*?"

"Doctor's orders."

So then she takes me into the shower. She gives me Phisohex

soap, and I had to scrub down from head to toe for about an hour. I think she was trying to kill some time. Because I'd no sooner come back out of the shower when I'd be bumming cigarettes again from Jackie and Mike. Or Robert. She was really down on the cigarettes. "If you're gonna go into major surgery, Mr. Hurley, you shouldn't be smoking!" I'd no sooner light up when she'd send me back in to scrub down again. It was like boot camp all over again! She'd say, "Mr. Hurley, you're not clean enough yet." And I'd say, "Well, you're not so swift yourself, toots." And she'd glare at me. "Get back in there and start washing."

This was about two in the afternoon. And suddenly I heard the gurney coming down the hall. Sarge comes in and says, "I think you'd better put the surgical gown on now." She and Robert put me into a surgical hat and surgical gown, very wrinkled, sterilized clothing. She shook it out, then helped me put it on.

And that's when I grabbed my cigarettes *and hid in the bathroom.* I did.

Sergeant Nurse yells out, "No, no, Mr. Hurley! The gurney is here for you. You have no time!"

"Like *hell* I have no time!"

And I *locked the door*!

I was really uptight. Nervous. *Terrified,* actually. A million things are running through your mind all at the same time. No one wants to go through an operation, no matter *what* kind it is. But believe me, there is no terror *on earth* as great as knowing that in the next fifteen minutes, *your heart is gonna be cut out of you!*

I finished two cigarettes. And they're knocking at the door. "Mr. Hurley!"

"Go away. I'm not ready yet."

Sergeant Nurse and Robert are *pounding* at the door. "Mr. Hurley, we're ready for you."

"That's nice, but I'm not ready for you yet!"

"Please come out, Mr. Hurley."

"I'm not done with my cigarette yet."

Sarge yells in, "What are you doing *smoking*? You're not supposed to be smoking! Put that cigarette out immediately! Mr. Hurley, do you hear me? Put it out at once! That's the worst thing you can do if you're going under is to have that cigarette!"

So I yell back out at them, "Listen—I've been on forty milligrams of Valium a day for the last three years! And today I ask for something to quiet my nerves down a little—and they give me *five* measly milligrams! For God's sake—they're gonna take me upstairs *to cut my bloody heart out*—and they give me five lousy milligrams! How am I supposed to feel? *How am I supposed to relax, for crissakes?*"

A minute later, one of the doctors comes to the door. "John, there's a long-distance call waiting for you at the nurses' station. You have to come out of there right away."

"Like hell I'm coming out. You're just saying that!"

"Please don't be difficult. You're being terribly immature about this whole thing, John. It's Dr. Kroner, calling long distance from New Jersey."

"That son-of-a-bitch! He'd get me about these cigarettes no matter *where* I am! He knew I've been smoking. He's got *radar*!"

"Come out, John."

"No."

"Come *out*, John. You can't hide in there forever."

I open the door. A blast of clean air hits me. I look around at everybody like I'm the condemned man about to go to the electric chair. I also expect everybody to grab me and put me into a straitjacket so I don't try any more escape and evasion tactics. But nobody makes a move. I walk out to the nurses' station and pick up the phone.

"Hello, Doc. It's me again. And I'm smoking."

"I have to call you long distance to hear that?"

We laughed.

"Have you been getting the pages of the journal I've been sending you?"

"Yes. I've got them all. The mail is pretty fast these days. I just wasn't expecting paper towels and napkins!"

"Can you read my handwriting?"

"I've been able to decipher it, yes. Listen John, I just want to wish you all the luck in the world. And all the best. I'm with you all the way, and the staff is keeping me posted. God be with you."

"Thanks, Doc. I'll be speakin to ya."

I hung up. Then I walked over to the gurney and lifted myself onto it, by myself. Ann took my hand.

I remember the ride up to the operating room. I was fully awake. We went down the hall to the elevator, then upstairs to the second floor. This is where the operating rooms are. Ann and I kissed each other good-bye, and they wheeled me inside.

I saw Dr. Shumway, the head surgeon, and the members of this surgical team. He looked over at me and nodded a greeting.

They strapped a mask over my face. I was in this preparation room just outside of the regular operating room, and pretty soon I don't remember anything else. Except that the mask felt like it didn't fit right. Someone put a needle into my wrist.

I was feeling stunned. Almost in a state of shock. That the whole thing had gone this far! I didn't know what was going to happen with this transplant. I figured, well, this is probably gonna be the end of me.

# 15

## The Surgery

*ANN* We just stood there.

On TV you always see them lifting somebody out of a bed. But John climbed onto the gurney himself. We all went up in the elevator with him and talked. Said everything was going to be OK.

Jackie kissed him. She said, "I'll see you in a little while."

And I kissed him. "Good luck, my darling."

And he said, "Yeah."

Mike shook his hand. "Good luck, John. See you later."

And they took him in.

The words were casual. But the impact on me I can never forget. As long as I live.

They closed the operating room doors, and they make such a horrible mechanical noise. They work on compressed air and close with a "swooosh!" Then they clank-locked shut. Tears started welling up in my eyes. I couldn't see John any more.

Jackie, Mike, and I looked for a nurse. But we couldn't find anybody. There wasn't a soul around. We saw a sign at one end of the corridor which said "Recovery Room. Waiting Room." So we sat around and waited. Mike disappeared after an hour, to go pick up John's sister, Joan, from the airport. He couldn't stand waiting at the hospital. Jackie and I walked around for a while. We had been told the operation would take from three to six hours. I was afraid to leave the floor. I'd seen a lot of people down at the other end, but it was all ICU.

After a couple of hours, Jackie went downstairs to the main floor and asked at the desk if she could find out how John was doing. She told the nurse on duty there that I was afraid to leave the floor where I was waiting. The nurse called directly upstairs to the operating room. She asked a few questions. Then told Jackie they were still working on him, but that everything was fine. No complications. He was coming along just fine. I don't know of any other hospital where you could do that, call directly to the operating room for information.

A half hour later there was a slight commotion in the hallway. First, a few doctors came by who I had never seen before; they were all perspired and tired looking. Then I see a nurse who I recognized. The minute she sees me, she comes running over. "Mrs. Hurley! Where have you been? We've been looking all over the hospital for you!"

"My God! Something went wrong!"

"No! Didn't anybody tell you they don't use this waiting room any more?" That's why we had been by ourselves! "Down at ICU is where you should have been waiting! The doctor is down there now for you."

We rushed all the way down to the end of the hall, and Dr. Stinson is waiting there for me.

"Mrs. Hurley. Everything has gone well. The operation was a complete success. And John is being stitched up right now. So far, everything is fine, and he'll be down within an hour."

Jackie and I embraced each other and just got hysterical crying. In fact we started to scream and jump up and down like a couple of crazy sorority sisters, screaming our heads off with joy, relief, and happiness that everything was over.

Jackie and I were with him when he first came out of the operating room. I wanted to hold his hand and touch him and tell him that it was a miracle, that he'd come through it with a new heart in him! It was a miracle. That's how I felt about it. That's what I kept telling myself. Jackie is shaking her head and she says the very same thing. "Ann, it's a miracle. It's truly a miracle. We've witnessed a miracle."

After they took him to his room, I went to a pay phone. I called my sister Barbara, and Janice got on the line.

"It's over. It's a miracle. He came through it fine. He's got a new heart beating in him."

I could hear the screams in the background. Neighbors and family were there, waiting to hear what happened to John. Our friend Jerry Wood fell backwards over a chair and almost fell down the stairs, he was so happy and had whooped so loud. The whole lake knew about it within an hour because the phone calls all started going out. It was phenomenal.

They put him into Room 203 of the Intensive Care Unit. It was like a small bedroom with TV and air conditioning. Monitoring equipment and all kinds of emergency equipment were on the back wall. Respirator. Defibrillator, oxygen, all kept covered and sterile. Plus an emergency surgery kit with instruments kept sterile there too.

They let me in to see him. Jackie stayed outside. He looked reasonably OK. The nurse said to me, "Talk to him, Mrs. Hurley. Try to bring him out of the anesthesia."

"John. This is Ann. John? It's Ann, darling. It's Ann. Can you hear me?" No response.

"John, honey. It's Ann. Can you hear me? You've had the operation. And everything is all right. Everything is all right, baby, and you have a new heart! It's a miracle, John. It's really a miracle. They did it. They gave you a new heart. And now you're going to be just fine again. You've come through it, darling. You've had the operation. It's over. And you're going to be just fine again. John? It's Ann. Can you hear me?"

And he stirred. It seemed as if he were trying to come out of it.

"John, honey, it's Ann. It's over. The operation is over. And it was a success, John. Isn't that a miracle? You've got a new heart!"

He stirred again. And I thought he was going to wake up. Instead, he brought his hands up, ran them over his chest, felt the bandages, and started to pull them off!

"My God. Nurse!"

She ran over at once and restrained him. "Talk to him some more, Mrs. Hurley. Tell him where he is."

"John! It's Ann. Do you know where you are? It's over. The operation is over! You're all right again John. It's Ann. John, you're in the hospital! John! Do you know where you are?"

And he shook his head no. Wouldn't answer. Just shook his head. No.

"Keep talking to him. Keep talking to him. Bring him out of it."

"John. It's Ann. It's me. Ann."

"Keep talking to him. Bring him out of it. Talk louder."

"John! Can you hear me? You're at Stanford. You're at Stanford! Do you know you've had a heart transplant?" I was almost shouting at him. "You've had a heart transplant! Do you know you've had a *heart transplant*?" He grabbed at his chest again, at the bandages, trying to tear at them. And he spoke for the first time.

"NO! NO! NO! NO! NO!" And he kept fighting the nurse. His eyes were still closed. "NO! NO! NO! NO! NO! NO! NO!"

I tried to reassure him. "John. It's Ann, honey. I called the children. They're so happy. And they send you all their love. Every one of them send you big kisses over the telephone. Janice and Joanie. And little John. Especially little John. He sent you an extra big kiss on the phone."

And now the tears started coming out of his eyes. So many tears. That I knew he could hear me. Or at least part of him could hear me and understand what was going on. And that's when I first noticed his hands getting funny. Like they were starting to get all crippled up. I showed them to the nurse.

"Don't you think his hands look a little peculiar? A little funny to you? They don't look quite right to me."

"No, Mrs. Hurley. That's only the anesthesia. That's nothing to worry about."

A doctor stopped by to write some notes on John's chart. I showed him John's hands.

"Don't they look a little funny to you, Doctor? Like they're a little crippled up?"

"I checked him thoroughly, Ann. And John doesn't look any different than any other transplant does who has just come from surgery. It's just taking him longer to come around. That's why he's not talking."

By this time, his sister, Joan, had gotten to the hospital. Jackie and I were waiting in the hall, walking back and forth, waiting for them to let us back in to visit him again. I met Joan as she stepped off the elevator. "Joan, it's all over. He came out of it fine!" And her knees sagged, she looked about to faint, and she started to cry.

I grabbed her arm. "Everything is OK! Perfect! John's perfect."

She was crying with relief, she was so happy. "Oh, thank God! Thank God! I was so worried! I was so worried!"

We went in to the nurse and I told her that his sister had arrived from Florida. "Can she go in and see him for a few minutes?"

She said, "Yes. But only for a very short time."

Joan said, "I understand. I'm a nurse."

She just got a look at him and came back out. "He looks well, Ann. He looks just fine. His color is good."

"Thank you, God. Thank you."

# 16

## The Vigil

*ANN*  There were two lives going in parallel here. John's. And mine.

I spent all my time at the hospital. When I got up in the morning, I showered, I dressed, and I went straight to the hospital. I ate my breakfast, my lunch, and my dinner at the hospital cafeteria, and I didn't leave until 10:00 at night. I'd call a taxi, go back to the motel, go to bed, set the alarm, go to sleep, wake up, get out of bed, and drag myself through the very same thing again. I had the feeling I was always tired and there wasn't anything I could do about it.

That first night, Jackie and Mike took a room next door, and stayed overnight. Joan moved in with me. The Ladners had thought to bring a bottle of Scotch and a bottle of vodka. Jackie said, "We don't know which you prefer, but it's for sure you need something. You've earned it!"

"So have you. All of you."

Joan said, "Amen to that."

So we all had a drink and sat back and tried to relax. Then Mike says, "Hey! It feels like the old days!"

"What do you mean, Mike?"

"I feel like I've just snuck three broads up the back stairway!"

After they left, I told Joan everything that had gone on for the previous week. She called her parents and told them everything was OK.

I took a sleeping pill.

The next morning—Sunday, November 17th—I went in, and his hands were much worse. All crooked and bent up out of shape. He looked like a vegetable. Just staring straight ahead.

I turned to the nurse. "Where's Doctor Copeland?"

"In his office, probably."

I found him and said, "There's something definitely wrong with him. I don't know how other transplants look or act, but I know my John, and I know his hands are severely crippled up, his eyes look very strange, and I just know there's something wrong with him."

"Mrs. Hurley, some people come out of the anesthesia differently than others. But if you'll feel better, I'll go in and look at him, and we'll have another doctor check him over too."

I waited in the hall outside his room for a half hour. Then they called me in.

"Mrs. Hurley. We think John has suffered a stroke."

"Oh, my God! What does this mean? How bad is it?"

"We think that either an air bubble or possibly a blood clot is affecting him. He may have gotten it coming off the heart-lung machine."

"But what are you telling me? Is John going to be all right?"

"We're not sure."

"But he's gonna come out of it? He will come out of this, won't he?"

"It's very hard to say, right now."

I guess I filled up and started to cry, and they said, "It's going to be all right, Mrs. Hurley. He's in no immediate danger. We'll watch him closely and see what happens."

"But how long could this take?"

"It could possibly take three or four months to pass. Or . . . and we have to be prepared for this . . ."

"Oh, my God! My God!"

"Just possibly . . . he might not come out of this at all."

"Oh Jesus . . . God!"

And then John started to move. And groan. Loudly.

*"UNNNNNNNN! UNNNNNNNNNN! UNNNNNNNN!"*

And he started to shake all over. His hands started trembling. His eyes went crazy and rolled back into his head like he was being electrocuted, and his mouth got crooked. His hands twisted up even further. They stiffened in a horrible way, and his whole body started writhing in spasms.

The doctors and the nurse started running around and got a tongue depresser and forced it into his mouth so he wouldn't choke. Then they held him down and gave him a shot of something. All this time they're shouting at me, to reassure me.

"He's just having a seizure, Mrs. Hurley. Don't worry. He's going to be all right. It's just a momentary seizure. Nothing to worry about."

I ran out of that room as fast as I could.

Seeing him like this was the most horrible torture anyone could have devised for me. The devil himself couldn't have created a worse torment for me. I tore the sterile gown off and threw it to the ground as their words kept sounding in my ear: "Nothing to worry about, Mrs. Hurley. It's just a seizure. Just a momentary seizure."

At that moment I knew that I was solely responsible for what had happened to him. And I wanted to die for it. I really did. Because I knew that I could have very easily talked him out of having the operation. We *knew* what the risks were. They told us that very plainly and clearly. We *knew* what they were and we went ahead anyway. I could have gone over his head and told the doctors I didn't want it done, that I was against it. And that would have been it. They never would have operated on him.

I ran into the ladies room, hysterical. My sister-in-law saw me in tears but kept her distance. She's very sensitive and wouldn't intrude. She stayed outside.

I wept bitterly. I blamed myself for having approved this operation, and now I'd made a vegetable out of him. And this was the *one* thing that John feared more than anything else in the world. More than death itself. To be helpless and enfeebled and completely dependent. And bedridden. It would be intolerable for him.

I was torn by three different feelings at the same time. I didn't know what I felt the most. I couldn't stop crying. My head was bursting. I was at once sorry for John, that he might be permanently left this way for the rest of his life. And at the same time I was sorry for myself, God forgive me, that I was going to have to live with him while he was in this condition. I was guilty for having done it to him—I knew it was all my fault—but at the same time, I wondered if God was punishing *him* for something he did!

Or was He punishing me?

I was so confused, I felt as if I were being torn apart in every direction.

A woman who had been in the ladies room when I entered came out of her stall, and, eyes averted, rushed outside, leaving me in there alone.

I came outside to the hallway about a half hour later. Joan was waiting there for me. She put her arm around me, to console me.

I suddenly felt very close to her. She held me and said, "It's gonna be all right, Ann. I know it will. I know it will. You just have to believe that." I said nothing. I didn't have the strength to speak.

"Ann, I don't know that much about transplants. But strokes ... and seizures ... they happen after an operation. It's a terrible thing to see, if you've never seen one before. It can be very frightening. And there could be some brain damage. We've got to be prepared for that. But Ann, they've been so honest and aboveboard about everything, and they've never held anything back ... that they'll tell you when something changes for the worse. If it does. And so far it hasn't. So please don't worry yourself sick over this. John's going to be all right."

Several hours later, they let us in to see him. He had all kinds of intravenous and wires and medications going into him.

"John. It's me, John. Ann. And Joan's here too, with me. Can you hear me? Can you hear me, John? Everything's going to be all right. The doctors say you came through the surgery beautifully and that they expect you to recover completely with your new heart. You're doing beautifully, baby. Just fine. And they're giving you medication and everything, and you're going to be up and walking around in no time. Can you hear me, John? And the children send their love."

And as soon as I said that, he started having another seizure. Just rippled over him. A bad one. And this time, he started pulling the intravenous and the wires out of his arm! His fingers started to cripple up again, and he clamped his hands around the tubes and wires, and his arms and hands were shaking so violently that he was beginning to cut himself pretty badly from the needles being torn out of his skin.

Thank God Joan was there! She forcefully untangled his fingers from the tubes and wires, wrestling him actually, while the nurse, who was there in an instant, was giving him a shot to quiet him down, and then putting a tongue depressor in his mouth.

Joan knew exactly what to do because of her training and experience as a nurse. She knew instinctively just how to react in the situation, and I admired her for staying so cool.

But when we came outside, Joan was shaken. "They're worse than I thought they were. I just thought he was having mild seizures. But these are serious."

We stayed very close to the hospital. I kept Jackie and Mike informed. Mike had returned to work, and Jackie had to take care of their children.

Dr. Copeland kept telling us, "No change."

We would go in every half hour. And several more times during the day he would have more seizures. They gave him shots, knocked him out, and afterwards he'd be exhausted. And wouldn't know anything. When he woke up, he'd continue to carry on whatever "conversation" or garbling he'd been having with you, without any memory of having had this seizure.

He would fade in and out of incoherency. One minute he'd say, "Ann. Want to go home. Ann. Want home. Go flying. Home." Next minute, he might be saying, "Car off. Buy it." He seemed to know me and Joan but couldn't carry on a normal conversation with us. He was very confused in his thinking. He couldn't feed himself. The nurses had to feed him. He couldn't hold the utensils properly. No coordination.

We were in and out the whole day. Dr. Copeland told us we could go home. "John is in no immediate danger, and if there's any change, I'll notify you immediately."

Joan agreed, saying, "We're close enough to the motel so that we can come back if we're needed. The doctor is right, Ann. You'd better go home and get some rest."

*Monday, November 18th.* I was up at 6:00 a.m. I woke Joan up, and we got to the hospital by 7:00, to start our visiting hours.

The seizures were worse. They were coming every hour. Then they hit every half hour. He was just going in and out of them constantly. He was restrained now, with leather straps, to keep from hurting himself or ripping anything out of his arm.

I called Jackie and Mike. They were there within the hour. We all just sat and looked at one another. It was like a death watch. And the nurses wouldn't let them in to see him. They were very strict about allowing only the immediate family in to see him.

Joan was very upset, and this worried me. "Ann, they're getting worse. They're coming too fast now. He's not getting any better. He could be in some danger now." She saw Dr. Copeland and went into a huddle with him. Then they came over to us.

"How is he, Doctor?"

"Mrs. Hurley, there's still no change. But we're going to bring in a brain specialist, to take brain-wave tests and see if there's any damage. And we have to get John on the breathing machines, to clear out his lungs before pneumonia sets in. We've got to build his lungs up."

"Pneumonia?"

"Don't worry, Mrs. Hurley. We're watching him closely."

As soon as he left, Joan went into John's room and looked through his records. Then she came out and sat down, looking grim.

"We'd better not leave the hospital."

"Oh, my God."

She was definitely alarmed. "When you're coming around from a stroke, the seizures start getting milder. They come less frequently. They don't get worse. But he's going in deeper—and they're coming more frequently than they should be—if he's really coming out of it."

Our vigil continued.

We watched them do the brain-wave tests on him. John was aware that something was going on. He seemed to be aware. But he didn't speak. Then they stuck little pins in his legs and feet. And it hurt him so bad he started to cry. But up until then, he hadn't been moving his legs. They were paralyzed from the stroke. And when they asked him to move his leg up and down, and move his toes, he couldn't. We weren't even sure if he understood what they were saying to him. He just lay there. Unable to move. After he stopped crying, he fell asleep.

John had hit bottom.

We went back to the motel.

*Tuesday, the 19th.* After more brain-wave tests, Dr. Copeland gave me the progress report. "There is no brain damage, Mrs. Hurley. Definitely no brain damage. I can assure you of that. Your husband's patterns are completely normal."

"Thank God. Thank God for that."

"But it very possibly could take six months before these seizures pass."

"Six months! How could he stand it? Will he be strong enough?"

"I don't think that's our primary concern at the moment. He's got to get that mucus out of his lungs. So we've got to get him to use the breathing machines and the blow bottles. We're going to need your help."

"Anything. Of course."

The one nurse that really brought him out of it was Inez. She was from Jamaica. She was fantastic. And afterwards, he swore to me she was the only nurse that he hated. "She tried to smother me. I swear, Ann, *she tried to kill me.*"

I said, "Inez? She's the one who *saved* you, if anyone did. She forced you to breathe with the breathing machine and blow bottles. The two of us were working on you for hours at a time!"

"Oh no. She was mean to me. I tell ya, she was a bitch!"

He was confused. The trouble started because he didn't want to use the breathing machine. He was refusing it. We had to hold his nose so he couldn't cheat and breathe through it, and avoid the machine. Inez held his hands, and we forced the mouthpiece into him.

I remember thinking to myself, "My God, I wonder what happens to the patients who don't have such supportive wives?" I wasn't being vain. I was being realistic. He was fighting Inez jamming this thing into his mouth. Every time he got it into his mouth, the machine would go PUFF! filling his lungs with air, so he could get rid of the mucus in his lungs and ward off pneumonia. It's set at a certain pressure, and PUFF! your lungs are filled, involuntarily. But he didn't understand it at all and was fighting it every step of the way.

The blow bottles are two bottles connected together. One of them has air in it, the other water. The principle is that you blow in one tube and move the water from one bottle to the other. Then the reverse. And this exercises your lungs, building their strength. At first, when we forced him to use it, he was so debilitated that it took at least *thirty* hard blows to move all the water from one bottle to the other. A month later, just to show how he began gaining his strength back, he could move all the water with *one* blow.

Later in the day, John had to sign a release form for another brain-wave test they wanted to do on him. A nurse just handed him the form, automatically, so that he could sign it. I was outside, in the hall. All of a sudden the nurse comes running out.

"Mrs. Hurley! Come quick! Your husband! Your husband! He's very upset! He's crying! You'd better come quick! He wants you right away!"

I rush in, and he's hysterical. Out of control. Nothing I could say would make him calm down. And then I realized what had happened. He had tried to write his own name. The pen was still in his hand. But he was unable to. He had forgotten how! *He had completly forgotten how to write his own name!*

The nurse and I tried to explain to him that after major surgery like this, it takes time to get back. But he was inconsolable. He thought it was all over for him. That he'd never be whole again.

"Ann, it's no use. It's no use. My mind is gone. My mind is gone."

"No John. No it isn't. This is just a temporary setback."

In a few hours, he calmed down enough to start practicing his writing. He was furious, really quite amazed actually, that he couldn't express himself in writing. He had papers, dozens of sheets, everything he could get his hands on, napkins, pads, tissues, practicing all the time with a pencil.

It took hours. But he never gave up. Never faltered. And once he got the "J," once he got the control for the "J" in John, it just came right back to him. At first it looked like a child's scrawl, but he just kept going over it and over it and over it. And finally he got there and was so proud he almost cried. Just for that name. John Edward Hurley. After that, and it took a full work day, it all came back to him.

*Wednesday, the 20th.* The seizures started to lighten up. They came every two or three hours. Then they started getting lesser and lesser, and finally, the nurse said, "He's really coming out of it, Mrs. Hurley."

Joan agreed he was doing much better.

Dr. Copeland stuck his head in the door. He had a surgical mask on and said, "How's John doing?"

I said, "You won't believe this—but John's holding his own dessert. He's feeding himself. Jell-O."

He takes one look and says, "I don't believe it! I'm seeing it, but I don't believe it!"

John was feeding himself. For the first time since the operation. Sort of like a baby would eat. His hands weren't right yet. So he was picking up his Jell-O with his fingers and putting it into his mouth. Like a child eats. Or a monkey.

Dr. Copeland says, "He's definitely coming out of it. Whatever was there is almost gone. It's just about passed through. If he has a good night, then he's got a good chance."

*Thursday, the 21st.* He wasn't completely alert yet, but he was well on the way back. The doctors were encouraged. They had never seen someone come back out of a stroke so quickly. I don't know if it was his will to live just fighting back, or his youth, or the bubble just passing through, or the blood clot dissolving, or what. But they were also very noncommittal about his chances for a full recovery. No guarantees. No time limit. They told me that these things are much too unpredictable. To be on the safe side, they decided to keep him on the medication they were giving him to control the seizures, for several more months. But they were firm in their prediction that the stroke posed no further danger. As far as dying was concerned.

I promised myself I'd have a nice nervous breakdown just as soon as I could arrange it. I deserved it.

Now that the seizures had stopped, John could talk again. He became fully conversant. I brought him up to date on everything. He couldn't get over the wonder of it all—that another man's heart was beating in his chest.

"Did they do it? Did they really put a new heart in me?"

"Yes, John. They really did."

"I can't believe it."

"I know. It's a miracle."

"I feel one thousand percent better, Annie. I really do. It's unbelievable! I feel terrific! It's like *magic* or something! *I'm a thousand percent better! It's a miracle! My God—it's a miracle!*"

# 17

## Hurley Power

**JOHN**  As soon as I could write again, I resumed keeping my journal for Dr. Kroner. I have a note in it saying, "Thurs. Nov. 21st. Got me out of bed and walked me across room. This was the first day they got me out of bed." The same orderly, Robert, helped me. Actually, he almost carried me out of bed, I was so weak. He's a big guy, and I was so limp that he had to pull me off the bed and walk me, physically, holding me under the arms and moving one of my feet at a time.

We didn't say anything. I was still pretty out of it, and he's a pretty quiet guy, and he just come over, got me out of bed, and held me. I was barely moving my legs. Couldn't support myself. But it was a great moment. To finally get out of that bed and feel like a whole man again. What a feeling!

And when he finally got me up and out of that bed, the first thing I wanted to do was take a crap!

"Robert, hey, do me a favor, will ya? Sit me on the commode over there, will ya?"

"Are you sure?"

"Yeah. I'm sure. I'm sure I'm sure."

There was this standing commode next to the bed. I hate them. They're such a pain in the ass! I've got a hangup I guess. I hate bedpans too! I never use them. Every time I'm hospitalized, and they try to pull that bedpan shtick on me, no sir! I *refuse*. That was the one thing I told the doctor. "No bedpan. Absolutely no bedpan! That's the one thing I won't go for."

"Why not?"

"Because even if it kills me, I'm getting out of this bed and going to that bathroom. Like a solid citizen."

So he ordered a special commode that looked like a chair, to be put next to the bed. Take a crap in bed? No way! You've got to draw the line someplace.

*Friday, November 22nd.* More journal: "EKG at 8:30 a.m., chest X-ray at 10:00. EKG at 3:00, X-ray at 4:00. Blood workup at 7:00. Got me out of bed and walked me across room to chair. Dragged me, actually. Thank God for Robert. He had me sitting up in a chair for a few minutes."

*Saturday, November 23rd.* It's one week after the operation.

They brought in a physical therapist. She was a very pretty young girl in her early twenties, with dark brown hair. She was about 5'6" and wore a blue pants suit made out of light nylon. Name was Jean. She showed me what exercises I had to do and brought in some dumbbells. Each one weighed one pound. And I couldn't lift them.

That afternoon I was allowed out of my room for the first time. I could only walk in the immediate hallway outside the ICU area. Jean was very nice and patient with me. Patience of a saint. After a few minutes in the hallway, she took me back to my room and started me off slowly with the dumbbells.

"When you feel yourself getting the least bit tired, don't overdo it, Mr. Hurley. Stop whatever you're doing."

What I was doing was trying to lift a one-pound dumbbell! And I couldn't lift it at all! She told me that after I was able to lift it, she'd give me a one-and-a-half pounder. Eventually I'd be able to work up to a *two* pounder.

"And then you'll be on your way again."

"Yeah. I know. Three, four, and *five*. Whoop-de-doo!"


*ANN*  The visiting hours in ICU were very limited. You were allowed fifteen minutes every four hours. Then for the next three hours and forty-five minutes, I'd be sitting in the waiting room. It's right outside the ICU section. So I did these jigsaw puzzles. Which aren't my thing. But after you've read all the current magazines and whatever paperbacks have been left lying around, there isn't much left to do.

Everybody waiting there was in the same boat. We were all going out of our skulls with worry and boredom. So to kill time, we made the puzzles a cooperative venture. Ten of us might be sitting around this large table, or on the floor. Some puzzles would have a thousand pieces. Some fifteen hundred. Some five thousand! And they're a real challenge!

"Oh my God, where does this tail belong?"

You'd sit there, looking and looking, and then get up, saying, "The hell with this goddamn thing! I never want to look at another goddamn puzzle again! I'm bored out of my skull, it's so crazy around here!" And someone would sit right down where you were doing it, and put the right piece in the right place. This went on for days.

Some people, like myself, stayed all day long. In fact, the guards at night, when they passed, they'd stop and put a couple of pieces in. The puzzles were pictures of scenery, flowers, stamps from around the world, and a *Playboy* centerfold of the Playmate of the Year.

The doctors never told me whose heart John had received. But I found out anyway. After the operation, this woman comes over to me, and we had talked the week before, while John was being evaluated. So I knew who she was, and she knew who I was. She motions for me to step off to the side so that she can tell me something private.

"What is it, Mildred?"

"I have something for you to see. Take a look at this."

And she hands me this newspaper that someone had left lying around. In it was an article about the donation of organs, and heart transplants in particular. And something rang a bell. It was about a young deputy sheriff, thirty-two years old, who had just died. His parents had donated his heart and other organs to Stanford. And the article said that heart transplant surgery had taken place November 16th, and that they could not divulge the name of the recipient, but that the surgery had been successful. The only reason that Mildred put two and two together was that we had been told that John was the only person who was to be given a transplant at Stanford that day.

# 18

## The First Acute Rejection

***JOHN*** Post-op entry in my journal, dated December 5, 1974: *"The first acute rejection of my heart took place 2½ weeks after the operation. I am still in Intensive Care. Somehow they didn't pick it up with my voltage readings."*

I've got ten clips in my heart. Look like the heads of a pin. They're actually implanted in my heart muscle, and placed at strategic locations. This is to detect rejections before they get too advanced or severe. As your heart is pumping blood through, the doctors are able to take electrical measurements from clip to clip. It gives them a reference by which to measure possible problems brewing without having to go in for a heart biopsy.

But they missed this one.

Fortunately I was scheduled for a routine heart biopsy. This is where they run a catheter tube into your jugular vein, and actually run it up inside a chamber of your heart. I watched the whole thing. You're awake when they do it. It's like a little clam shovel. They take tiny snips of tissue out, then pull the catheter out, and drop the tissue into a specimen jar. The examination of this tissue, which they then slice into hundreds of tiny pieces, revealed that I was just about to have an *acute* rejection.

They caught it at precisely the moment it was just starting. So they administered ATG shots right away. That night. They call them rabbit shots. It's a vaccine made from rabbit thymus. Very potent and exotic stuff. Has to be stored frozen solid. You get it in the tops of your thighs. You're in your room, and the nurse administers them. The first thing she does is put heating pads on your legs for about half an hour. And you're not allowed to move. Then she gives you a mild pain-killer. And a tranquilizer to relax you.

Then she starts the injections. And they hurt like *hell.* Even going *in* they hurt. You've never gotten a needle like this in your life! My God! The sweat starts *pouring* off you. It's *agony.* You feel like someone has just taken a baseball bat and hit you five times as hard as they could possibly whack you, across your legs. That's how strong this stuff is. Torture.

Then I got sleeping pills. I would have welcomed *heroin* at that point.

Father John Hester comes into my room and introduces himself. "Mr. Hurley, I hear you're a Catholic. My name is John Hester."

I look up at him. He's tall, around thirty-eight years old, and wearing a regular priest's outfit with the white collar. He had a real comfortable-looking face. He made me feel relaxed and at ease with him, right away.

"Would you like to receive Communion?"

"Yes, Father. I would."

We got to talking, and finally he says, "Tell me, what do you think of all this, anyway?"

And I say, "What do you mean?"

"Well, you've just been given someone else's heart. You've had a transplant. Do you have any hangups about it? Any bad feelings on your mind? With religion?"

I guess he wanted to know what my feelings were, and if I thought maybe I had done something wrong, as far as the Church was concerned, by extending my life instead of going when my time was supposedly up. And I said, "Truthfully, Father, I think it's a miracle. I really do. To me, it's remarkable! It's one of the rarest things that I have ever heard of being done. A couple of weeks ago, they rushed me out here on a plane. I couldn't breathe; I could hardly speak; I was panting; I was out of breath. Look at me now!"

"It truly is a miracle. I know what you mean."

"But the thing that I don't understand about this whole thing, Father, is that—I once worked in Puerto Rico, and when I was down there, I was in an automobile accident which by all rights should have killed me. I ran right into the back of a solid steel milk truck. Completely demolished my car. Totally. But nevertheless, I got up, and walked away from it. Just walked away. The car was so bad that the whole dashboard was wrapped around me. Slivers of glass in my arm. But nothing really happened to me. And when I was transferred back to the States, I totaled more cars, and I walked away from those, and nothing happened. And here I am. Now I've had this massive coronary. I never thought I was gonna live. The doctors had written me off. I was told before this transplant that I had maybe two weeks more to live, and here I am today. They found a donor, and just look at me. Aside from a few complications, I feel terrific! *And that's the part I don't understand!*"

So he said to me, "John, you've got to remember that *everybody* is put on this earth to accomplish something. We all have a fate and a destiny. Apparently, whatever you've been created for, you haven't yet accomplished."

## The First Acute Rejection

"OK, Father. I'll tell you what. You know . . . I have never been a religious man. I've been a *faithful* man. I believe in God. But I have never been an extremely religious type of a man. So that means that you're a lot closer to that guy upstairs than I am. That's for sure. So do me a favor, will you, Father? When you find out just what that man upstairs has created me for to accomplish, you let me know just as fast as you can. Will you do that for me, Father? Because when I know what it is, I'm *not gonna do it*!"

Well, he looked at me and didn't know what to say. He just sat there for a minute, digesting. It had to sink into him. Then all of a sudden, he breaks out into a giant-sized smile that lit up that room, and laughed out loud till it hurt both of us.

They nipped this rejection in the bud.

While you're recuperating, you're all by yourself. There's really nobody to talk to except the nurses. Which can be interesting. But after a while, they all look the same, because, with all the garb they've got on, only their eyes are exposed. Sometimes one of them would bend over and she'd have a real short skirt on, and I'd think to myself "This is gonna be a very interesting day. Maybe I'll throw *pennies* on the floor!"

But you always had a different nurse. Every day. There were 120 Intensive Care nurses. And wearing all that garb in there, it gets hot as hell. They've got to wear what Ann's got on, mask, gloves, booties. Something for the hair. It was a rough tour. So they looked forward to their breaks.

But someone was always in there with me. Always. They never left me alone. Not even for a second. You'd hold conversations with them, but you don't know them, and they don't know you, so you're sort of manufacturing questions and answers, and they're doing likewise. "Where are you from? Do you have any children? Are you married? How old are you? How long have you been in California?"

And of course, when they came in, they'd always ask me the same questions. "When did you have your original heart attack? What do you do for a living? How long did it take to find a donor?"

So to me, it was repetitive.

And I wasn't getting any sleep. I'd just about fall asleep, and they'd be waking me up to give me more pills. Around the clock. I told one of the nurses about it. "I'm not getting any sleep at all!" And she showed me her notebook. She had already written in it, "What John needs is some sleep. Leave him alone!" I blew her a kiss. She winked at me.

The thing was, you had no privacy. None whatsoever. You're never left alone. My bed was in the corner. The nurse's little table-desk was a few feet away, off to one side, and on the other side was a sink, a cabinet for my medications, the defibrillator (that I was petrified at the sight of), and the oxygen and breathing apparatus. There were no curtains to pull around you. The nurse would be in there, writing her reports, so you'd have a woman in there twenty-four hours a day.

You're trapped in that room. Frustrating as hell. You want to do something. Anything. But what can you do? Watch television? Where they have soap operas on, and quiz shows, and all this other garbage? So you'd want to read a book or a magazine, and you'd pick it up and if I got through a *page,* it'd be a lot. *Reader's Digest, Field & Stream, Golf Digest, The Wall Street Journal.* Everything was a complete blur. Because one of the immunosuppressive drugs they were giving me was Prednisone. And one of the side effects is blurry vision. For a while, until my system got used to it, I could hardly read. And couldn't see to write at all.

## The First Acute Rejection

At first, I couldn't even read the letters we got from the children. Ann would have to read them to me. The drug affects the muscles of your eyes. But I got used to it. The kids kept in touch by sending pictures, tape cassettes, and letters. I couldn't help it, but I cried whenever I heard from them. I missed them so much.

> Dear Daddy, We miss you very much. We think of you all the time, and pray you're feeling better and can come home soon. Love and XXXXXXXXXXXX, Janice, Joan, and John.

Any letter that came from them I'd hold in my hands for hours at a time.

I was down to 147 pounds, from 195 when I came out to California. I looked like Halloween. Ann said, "You look terrific, John! What are you complaining about? You'll put it back on." But there was nothing left. A guy 6'5" just skin and bones. My legs and arms were just hanging. I had no ass. When I sat, I sat on two bones.

I was famished all the time because of the medication, and because the doctors put me on a 1000-calorie diet.

You're *absolutely* famished. If someone were to take something off my tray while I was still eating, I'd put a fork right through their hand! Really. ZAP! So I'd be very selective (and very limited) as far as what my choices were. Then they come in with the tray, and half of what you ordered has been left off of it! I used to get so mad, I thought I'd blow a fuse. After a while, I learned how to control my fury, and I wouldn't let the person who delivered my meal get out of the room until I checked with my menu, and then what was on my tray, to make sure that every single *scrap* was there!

I noticed so many discrepancies, I started sending little notes down to the chef.

Dear Chef: This morning you left off my white toast. Therefore, and with malice aforethought, I hope a camel with weak kidneys backs into your breakfast table, to start off your day the way you've started off mine! Sincerely, John E. Hurley.

You really become a wild man. Food becomes an obsession. But nothing changed. I went hungry.

For example, I'd order an egg for breakfast. And I'd ask to have it "over light." And I'd get the egg—and it would be just laid out on a plate, *floating* there, the white not cooked at all. It was *Yugggggh!* And I'd lift the cover off that tray and just look down at it—and want to throw it across the room. Other times, if I ordered a hard-boiled egg, they'd take the *yolk* out of it! All you had laying there was the empty white container part. *The yolk was taken completely out of the egg!*

So I wrote more notes to the chef. I used to say, "What's the point? Don't give it to me! Don't serve it at all if this is all I'm going to get! I'm not some prisoner of war!"

After a few weeks, they moved me from Intensive Care, to what they call a "Self-Care" type of a unit. It's in an adjoining wing. Again, you're isolated in your own room, but the precautions, while strict, are not as strict as before. Self-Care is a training program, to get you ready for life outside the hospital. They teach you to take your own stool samples, to see if you have any blood coming through because of internal bleeding (because you're on blood thinners all the time).

Every single time you move your bowels, or urinate, you've got to test yourself. You have to measure your intake and output of fluids, to see if you're building up fluids and sugars within your body. You have to chart everything down. Specifically—what time you took your pills, which ones they were, what the results of the stool test were, what the urine test showed, how much water you took in. They give you standard-size cups, marked in cc's, so you can keep a constant record. To this day I have to do these tests. Without fail.

Self-Care training also makes you very cautious against doing anything that will expose you to infection. So if you were walking in the hospital, you'd automatically avoid the wards with contagious diseases. Or outside, you wouldn't go to a movie on opening night, with a mob of people there. You'd wait a few weeks until business tapers off. Or go to a drive-in. You wouldn't go to zoos. Go to an early mass, like at 6:00 in the morning.

Father John had a small portable refrigerator, which he lent to me. Three foot by three foot in size. He and Ron Glass, the EKG technician, moved it into my room. And I kept beer in it. I was allowed to have two beers a day. Always had Coors. Used to serve it to visitors in Styrofoam coffee cups. We kept quite a few six-packs in stock.

The first beer of the day was delicious. I used to look forward to it, dream about it, start dreaming about it the night before! The nurses had to clean the cans off with alcohol to prevent infection, before I could pour the beer out into my glass. There were many times I felt like having two beers in the morning. Because after the first, the second one usually tastes even better.

*ANN*  I met Janice at the airport. My sister-in-law Joan had returned to Florida after John was out of danger. Janice embraced me and immediately asked, "How's Daddy? How's Daddy?"

We went directly to the hospital.

Outside of John's room there was a cabinet, and they had a list of how visitors were to put everything protective on. First, you washed your hands with Phisohex. Then you put your gown on, then your booties, your hat, your mask, and your gloves. Everything was this disposable paper, except for the gown, which was a regular surgical gown. Everything was right there in each drawer, and you just took out what you needed. You got used to this routine after a while, and when you came out, you disposed of the whole thing.

And for when John wanted to see the nurses' names, there was a big roll of tape, and a marking pen. So I tore off a big piece, wrote "I AM YOUR WIFE ANN!" on it, and pasted it across my chest. Janice laughed and said, "That's telling him!" Then she tore off a piece and wrote "I AM YOUR DAUGHTER JANICE!" And pasted it across her chest.

We went in to see him. He looked up and at first didn't know who we were because we were all covered up. Then he managed to catch sight of our name tapes.

"What? I'll be a—"

Janice rushed over to him and threw her arms around him. "Daddy! Oh I'm so glad to see you! I'm so glad to see you!"

They both started crying and held each other tightly.

"I'm glad to see you too, honey! I'm so glad to see you too! You look wonderful! How was your flight? Oh, you look wonderful, darling! Just wonderful!"

"So do you, Daddy! I'm just so glad to see you!" She was relieved to see both of us again, and to see that her father was OK. "I'm so glad to see you, Dad. I missed you so much!"

"I missed you too, honey. But we're together now, and that's the main thing."

I went over to them and put my arms around both of them. "We're all together now, thank the good Lord."

# 19

## Out of the Hospital

*JOHN*  It was getting toward the middle of December, and the doctors decided to allow me out of the hospital on a brief pass. Before I went out the door, I asked Dr. Copeland if the mask was really effective in keeping out germs. He said, "The effectiveness is there, to a degree. To what degree, we really don't know. It depends on what kind of germs are lurking about. But it works *two* ways. Because people take one look at you with it on and think you have a communicable disease. So they stay the hell away from you!"

It's true. They stare at you. Especially kids. They sort of are amazed at this masked person walking the hallways. But at Stanford, anyone who had a mask on was a transplant. It was a telltale sign. You'd hear people whispering, "There goes a transplant."

The first time I stepped outside of the hospital, I saw how really beautiful the grounds and buildings are. And the air! My God. It was fantastic! You couldn't believe it how it feels to get fresh air after being confined for such a period of time. Just nice, cool, refreshing air. And the air had an *aroma*. Maybe it was the mask. It always had the aroma of a fireplace burning. You know, the smoke from the wood? Plus, it was fresh.

Ann was there, Janice, our friends Etta and Lincoln Blakely, and Fred and Helen Kelly. We took some snapshots out by the fountain, in the front. It was gorgeous. Then we got into Fred's car and went over to H. Salt.

H. Salt is a franchise place, like Arthur Treacher's Fish and Chips here. I had to keep my mask on, to avoid infection. It was an absolute requirement of my pass. So we go into this place and are waiting up front at the counter for our fish and chips, and I'm sorta standing in the background. I'd been told to avoid crowds. Now, they've got one of those TV surveillance cameras panning the room, watching out for trouble. And I'm standing there, not on line, because I can't eat these rich, greasy, batter-dipped foods. I'm just standing there with my mask on.

Well, the next thing I know, some guy from security comes walking into the place, with the uniform and walkie-talkie, and sidearms. And he's looking at me with the mask on. He thought I was gonna hold up the joint. Either that, or he thought I'd just escaped from some home for the criminally oddball. He's got his hand on his pistol, ready for me to make my move. Ready for anything. Then he goes over to the manager, never once taking his eyes off me, and he and the manager have a little conference. Fortunately the manager put two and two together, and must have seen earlier transplants, so he explained the situation to the guard, and the man leaves, still eyeing me up and down. I took a deep breath and relaxed.

After the H. Salt experience, if we were going out to a restaurant, we'd call ahead of time, make reservations, and explain I was a heart transplant. We'd ask to be seated way out of the direct path of where the people would be entering the restaurant, and preferably in a corner where there was some ventilation and where I wouldn't have people marching back and forth near my table. In fact, you could even request that they prepare your meal without salt, and make sure you only got margarine instead of butter. Just by phoning ahead. The restaurant managers were very nice about it. Very cooperative. Because this was the Palo Alto area near Stanford, so they knew.

Christmas Eve.

I wanted to go to a good restaurant with Janice and Ann. The fella who did the EKGs in the hospital, Ron Glass, his father was a chef at the Regency Hyatt House. He set all the reservations up for us. We had a terrific dinner. Even if I did have to walk into the place looking like the Lone Ranger. I think I had the biggest prime rib steak I've ever eaten in my life, a couple of martinis before it, and a bottle of the driest wine with it. Superb!

Janice really enjoyed herself, too. She ordered a whole Maine lobster. But they didn't have lobster on the menu. So she had steak as well.

Then I put my mask back on, and we went back to my Self-Care room. I still was not an outpatient yet. We called home. Little Joan spoke to us first.

"What did Santa bring for you, Joanie?"

"I gotta baby-alive doll!"

"What's that, Joanie?"

"A baby-alive doll! You feed her real food and then she messes her diaper!"

"That's terrific, Joanie! Did you get anything else besides your baby-alive doll?"

"Yes."

"What?"

"I got an umbrella doll-carriage-stroller for it, too."

"What's that, Joanie?"

"It's a stroller, with an umbrella over it."
Then little John got on.
"I got a new tool set, Daddy!"
"Oh? That's wonderful, John. What's in it?"
"Everything."
"Everything? What's everything?"
"It's got a saw in it. And a hammer. And a screwdriver!" And I'm thinking to myself, Oh, Jeez, wait until he gets home and starts working on the legs of the furniture!
"Bye, Daddy!"
"Bye, John."
Then Bobbie and Ronnie got on and we wished them Merry Christmas. We thanked them again for taking the kids, and asked them how they were getting along. Ronnie had been sick himself for a while, but things were under control. They asked how Janice was behaving.
"Is everything all right with Janice?"
"Sure. She's just fine."
"Great. You sound pretty great yourself, John."
"I'm feeling pretty good, all things considered."

We exchanged gifts in my room. Janice gave me a sweater, shirt, and slacks, a whole outfit. And I had made a pair of moccasins for her in physical therapy. She was surprised that I had made them myself. Ann bought herself a blouse and a pants suit as a Christmas present from me, since I wasn't allowed out yet on a regular basis. She thanked me for them. Then, like any other evening, at ten o'clock it was lights out, and Ann and Janice had to head back to the hacienda.

As a Christmas present, I bought Dr. Copeland a bottle of champagne, and Ron Glass a bottle of wine. But for Father John, I bought him something special. A bottle of Blue Nun wine!

Father John came around quite often, even though he was extremely busy. He covered a children's home, and two or three other hospitals as well as Stanford. He was a very consoling type of a person. He'd hold a small mass in my room and give me Communion. He'd say a prayer and lead me through other prayers. Ann was generally there, and on occasion so was Janice and my sister, Joan. Then, in his own words, he'd come out with a prayer, and bless me and the family, that everything was gonna be all right. Then he'd serve us Communion and give us the Host.

He was also very humorous. Always had a story to tell about some incident he'd encountered. Like for example, it seems that there was a woman in the hospital, in her seventies, and she was very ill. I don't know if they expected her to live or not. But she and this elderly man had fallen in love. And they wanted to get married. Right away. So Father John asked her, "What faith are you?" Turns out they weren't Catholic. "Well, do you have the marriage license, blood certificates, and . . .?" They put their hands up to stop him from continuing. Apparently they didn't have any of those things yet. And she was a wheelchair patient.

So Father John got together with all of the nurses, and told them about the engaged couple who wanted to get married. They all agreed to help out. In order to decorate the chapel for the wedding, Father John and the nurses *hijacked* these big carts that used to come around and drop off all the plants and flowers that came in for patients in the hospital. They took all the cards off the plants, brought them to the chapel, and decorated the chapel beautifully. So beautifully, that it looked like a royal wedding. Then the nurses found a gown for this woman. God only knows from where.

So with twelve hours' notice, they had the gown—and decorated the chapel with flowers that belonged to every other patient in the hospital! Then they had the kitchen cook up a small wedding cake, and someone brought in a bottle of champagne, so that after the wedding, everybody would have their wedding cake and champagne!

And as soon as the ceremony was over, and the bride and groom had left the chapel, the nurses took the cards and just stuffed them back in the flower arrangements. At random. They had no way of knowing which ones belonged to which. Then they delivered them to the patients. People who were sent a dozen red roses wound up with cactus plants and *ferns*!

But that was Father John. A wonderful man.

When you're in isolation, your door is closed all the time. I knew the man next door was in trouble and having a problem. He'd been operated on after me. There were three of us transplants up there at the time. This young boy, Patrick Sherlock, who was fifteen, and this older gentleman, and myself. I knew something was going wrong for the older guy because when I would be walking up and down the hallway, they had voltage readings posted for each of us, daily, and you could see that his voltage was just coming down, down, down, and down. Every day. Plus I knew there was a lot of activity, doctors going in and out of his room all the time.

The nurses had decorated our doors, really beautifully, for Christmas, with all kinds of tinsel and ornaments, and on this older gentleman's door they had made a picture of him looking like Santa Claus. A caricature. Very nice. They drew Santa but included his own personal features, like the glasses he wore. And around his feet they had rabbits, to signify the ATG rabbit shots they were giving him, to fight the rejection.

So I come out one morning, going down to X-ray about 7:00 a.m., and all of a sudden I see his door is wide open. And they had also taken down all the Christmas decorations. And the room is empty. And the bed was stripped. I just walked by. I knew. Instinctively I knew what had happened.

I went down, had the X-rays taken, came back up, and was in my room eating a poached egg when Ann came in.

"Ann, do me a favor. Go out and see if they've posted the voltages." So she goes out, comes back in, and says, "Yes. Yours is OK." So I say, "What's the guy's next door?" And she said, "There is none for him." I said, "I don't think he's there any more." She looked at me for a long moment. Then she said, "He died. I knew about it. I just didn't want to get you upset."

There's a grapevine there among the transplants. The news spreads very fast. If you don't see someone when he's supposed to be there, you ask, "Where is so-and-so?" From week to week it would vary. Generally something was occurring with one of them. One guy developed diabetes and went into a coma. Another guy developed a lung infection. Another guy broke out with cancer on his hands.

My reaction was not so much a shudder of fear as a realization that this could happen to *me*. They explain to you that you've got to watch out for infections and not expose yourself to this or that. It's sort of a realization—when you see all of these top doctors trying to keep this guy alive, and then to see him pass away anyway, despite their best, sometimes even heroic, efforts, you know exactly what they're talking about. It enlightens you that they're not kidding, they're not fooling around. It's no joke.

Ann and I were walking to physical therapy this one morning, and we're walking down the hallway on the other side of the hospital where they did a lot of research and autopsies and pathology. Ahead of us there's this colored guy orderly, pushing a corpse on a wheeled table. And the stiff's not covered up. The orderly sees us coming and he *knows* I'm a heart transplant, and I don't know what was going through his mind except "I'ze got to get the hell *outta* here with this body so's dah white man don't see it!" And every door he's trying to open, to wheel this body out of our sight, is locked! He's running from *door* to *door* trying to get this thing out of my way so I wouldn't be exposed to the sight of it! I felt embarrassed for him. He finally just *stood* there with his arms outstretched, trying to shield our gaze from this stiff any way he could. Ann and I broke up.

I kept pushing. I told the doctors that I wanted to be discharged as an outpatient by New Year's Eve. And I sort of used a little reverse psychology on them. I'd keep pushing and pushing. Now they don't like to give you any false hopes. But I kept saying, "I'll be outta here by then. I'm feeling very good." I'd sort of give them a week *earlier* than the date I would like to get out. And Dr. Copeland was giving me two weeks *later* than the date he wanted to see me discharged. So it was sort of worked out as a compromise. New Year's Eve became an ideal opportunity. I said, "You know, Dr. Copeland, it would be so nice to be released on New Year's Eve. December 31st. Around noon. Through the *front* door. And be able to spend it with my wife and daughter, in our own apartment."

So I was released on New Year's Eve. Through the front door. I went *out* first class! It was a great feeling. I was just looking forward to spending the night in my own bed, a double bed, instead of a hospital bed! And to have the freedom to walk around. And not be tied down any more.

The first thing we did on the way home was do some grocery shopping. Then we stopped at a liquor store and picked up some booze, wine, champagne, beer, and a corkscrew. I wanted a martini so badly I could taste it!

There's a three-hour time differential between out there and the east, so at nine o'clock that night we were watching the Guy Lombardo show taking place in New York, with the ball coming down at midnight in Times Square. Janice was asleep already, so it was just Ann and me watching Guy. And that was our New Year's Eve.

At midnight, our time, the phone rings, and it's Janice's friends from New Jersey calling (3:00 A.M. their time). They woke us up. I could have strangled them.

"Hello. Mr. Hurley? Hey! How ya doin'?"

"Fine. Who is this?"

"It's Kevin."

"Kevin who?"

"I'm a friend of Janice's."

"Oh."

"Hey! Happy New Year, huh?"

"Yeah. Happy New Year."

"Can I speak to Janice? Linda, Ellen, and Colleen are with me too."

"Yeah, sure. I'll get her. Hold on."

I turn to Ann, who is rubbing the sleep out of her eyes. "Would you get Janice? It's her friends on the phone, calling to wish her Happy New Year."

She looks at me and says, "Terrific."

Ann goes into Janice's room and wakes her. A moment later, Janice comes into our room, plunks herself down on our bed and picks up the phone. A two-way coast-to-coast coffee klatch begins.

"Hey! Hiya Kevin! Hey! Hiya Linda, and Ellen. And hey! Colleen! How are ya? Yeah I'm fine. We're doin' real good. Hey! Happy New Year to you guys too! It's really nice of you to call! What time is it there? Really? Three o'clock? Yeah! It's midnight here! Yeah. Real good! Real good! Super! Um-hmm! Super! Real good! Yeah, right. Right! No kidding! No kidding? No kidding! No! Yeah? No! No! I don't believe it! No! No! Yeah? No!"

A half an hour later it was over. Ann and I grumped back to sleep.

New Year's Day we went to an Italian restaurant that we found. The people who owned this place were from Paterson, New Jersey. And it was a gold mine. They called it "Frankie, Johnny, and Luigi, Too." That was the name of it. There were lines around the block. And they had the most delicious pizza on this *planet*.

I'm wearing my mask, and I step up to the counter, and the kid there takes one look at me and almost drops his drawers. In a real shaky voice, a stutter almost, he says to me, "Y-y-y-yes?"

"I'll have six slices, please, the regular, no sausage. And three Seven-Ups. To go."

"Y-y-y-es, sir!"

We're standing there, and all the kids are poking their parents in the ribs, saying, "Look, Dad! Looka that guy! He's weird isn't he?" And the parents are shushing them, whispering, telling them to be quiet and stop staring at me.

One little colored kid, he just pipes up, "Hey man, whatchoo got that mask on yo' face for? You sick or somethin'? Man, you a real *weird* dude!"

So I turned to him and said, "You know what? I'm a heart transplant. I've got a brand new heart inside my chest."

He looks up at me and says, "No *shit*?"

# 20

## Anchored to the Clinic

**JOHN** After New Year's, the three of us began our day-to-day living. We'd get up in the morning and wonder where we were going and what we were gonna do. And was it a clinic day?

We lived around the clinic. You couldn't go too far from it. We had invites from our friends to go down to Los Angeles, and there were a lot of places that we wanted to see. But, come Monday and Thursday, I had to report to the clinic for tests. Like clockwork. So we did as much sightseeing within a hundred mile radius as we could.

We lived at number 184 of the Brookside Apartments. On Rainbow Drive, in Mountain View. It was recommended to us by the father of this fifteen-year-old boy who had a heart transplant, Patrick Sherlock. It was just gorgeous. Beautiful layout. It was in a complex of two-story buildings.

You walk into a main entrance lobby which really looks plush. Wall-to-wall red and black shag carpeting in the reception room, and in the recreation area there were a couple of pool tables, a

Ping-Pong table, a tremendous-size sitting room where you could watch television, and a kitchen so you could reserve the room and have a cocktail party if you wanted. Walk outside of that, and you're in a big courtyard with all the apartments overlooking, and a little brook running through it. And there was a small lake on the grounds, with fish in it, a swimming pool, a sauna, a Jacuzzi whirlpool bath, and their own professional laundry.

We only wanted a one-bedroom apartment, but all they had left was a three-bedroom. We took it.

California is very tranquil. Except for the freeways. And nobody ever has to dress for appearance's sake. The only thing you have to have on if you enter a restaurant is *shoes.*

We played miniature golf. Went to Marine World. Drove over to Santa Cruz and had lunch on the ocean pier. Just about every day we'd go someplace. If it was a rainy day, I'd stay home and work on my newest hobby, decoupage.

We'd take rides to the foothills, and generally for lunch we'd find one of these fast food franchise places. I'd avoid anything greasy. Which wasn't easy. Ate more bread than hamburger. Or we'd pack a picnic lunch. The foothills are actually quite high and, in the wintertime, get snow on their peaks and tips. Just gorgeous. The most beautiful scenic views. We took a lot of Instamatic pictures up there.

The farthest we went was Pebble Beach. And Carmel and Monterrey, and the Seventeen-Mile Drive, which is maybe 150 miles from the hospital. Ann wanted in the worst way to see this Seventeen-Mile Drive because all her friends at the hospital and everybody she met had all been raving, "You've got to see this Seventeen-Mile Drive! It's so beautiful, you've got to see it before you leave!"

We argued all the way down there. I didn't want to go. But

when I got there, I loved it. You'd see the seals laying on the rocks, sunbathing and swimming and making one hell of a racket! They have seals right in the ocean. Loaded with seals. And I was amazed to see a golf course nearby just loaded with deer. Tame deer. I'd see the guys hit the ball and almost have to chase the deer away.

If I had had my choice I would have stayed out in California.

On Monday and Thursday, the clinic days, there were certain times set aside just for heart transplants, so that all their tests can be done and finished as early as possible in the morning. To avoid crowds.

On an average, there were ten of us. We all talked to one another, to find out how everybody was doing and feeling. And mostly we talked about food. Like how to fix a good drink without too many calories! Wishful thinking! Or where you could buy this breakfast sausage that was really terrific, meaning low in cholesterol and fats. These guys, a lot of them would do their own cooking. Prepare their own meals without salt. Get as much fat off of meats as they could. Some of them, of course, would cheat. And it would show up right away on the scale.

Their ages ranged from fifteen to twenty-three, later thirties like me, early forties, and a few in their fifties. It wasn't a nervous crowd at all. We all had something in common.

First thing you did when you came in was get on the scale and weigh yourself. And this was amusing when you watched the other guys. First of all, they'd wear as light a clothing as possible. Some of them would even empty their pockets before they got on the scale. Some would take off their shoes.

Then you wrote your name on the blackboard, and what time you checked in. Then you went to where they took your blood from you. It was almost like a butcher shop, where you'd have to take a number and wait your turn.

After that, you'd go down to X-ray and have your films taken. Then you could eat (because up till now you weren't allowed to, before your blood test). We would go to the cafeteria and have a cup of coffee and a piece of grapefruit. Then we'd go upstairs and we'd gather in the EKG room. My pal, Ron Glass, was the technician.

And this was sort of the moment of truth. This is where you find out what your voltage is. If it's up, it's good. But if it was down, you might be having a rejection problem. That's the telltale sign. If it was down, they would have to do a heart biopsy on you. No one looked forward to that. If they found it *was* a definite rejection, they'd readmit you, and increase your Prednisone. And if that didn't start to bring up your voltage, they'd give you these ATG rabbit shots. God forbid.

After we finished our EKGs, we'd wait in the waiting room —to be called by the doctor in the sequence in which we signed in in the morning. After he examined you and adjusted your medication dosages if necessary, you'd go to the nurse, and give her your prescription order, if any. Then you'd go down to the pharmacy, pick up the prescription, and you'd be free for the rest of the day.

They took X-rays of me every clinic day. As part of the routine. And one day, after several weeks as an outpatient, they discovered a shadow on my lung. Two visits later, the shadow became more pronounced. So they readmitted me to the hospital, because they were alarmed and wanted to find out what it was. They thought it might be an infection brewing, or worse, and if it was—because of the immunosupressants you're on, it can overtake you in twenty-four hours, and you can *go,* just like that. So they gotta catch it right away.

So they readmit me, and the shadow was in such a position

that it was awkward to perform what they call a lung biopsy, where they go into your lung and draw out a specimen from where the infected area is and culture it, to identify it and determine what antibiotic they can give you to fight it.

But with me, I developed this spot so close to the aorta that at first they didn't know how to approach it. I was on blood thinners, and this meant that if they were to go in with a needle and accidentally puncture the aorta, which is a major artery, forget about it. You're finished, right there. They weighed the consequences. If they didn't go in and find out what it was, it might spread, and the end result would be the same.

So after a large consultation with two groups, the surgeons and the general staff, they decided to go in with this needle and do a biopsy. First of all, they explained to me what the chances were and had me sign releases. They fully explained to me just how dangerous a procedure this is, and I released them from all liability. I never read a damn thing. I just felt—*sign* it, or don't have it done. An Italian-looking chunky technician explained everything to me.

"John, when they go in there, there's a one-third chance of your lung collapsing. Which we can take care of right away. That's no problem."

"No problem? My lung collapsing? No problem?"

"No problem. Then there's a one-third chance of nothing happening to you whatsoever. We'll get the biopsy, and everything will be fine."

"Fine."

"Fine. No problem. The procedure has to be done while we're looking at your insides through a kind of fluoroscope machine that gives living X-rays of your insides, as it's happening. But there's a certain amount of distortion."

"Distortion? What do you mean, distortion?"

"Well, I mean it's like as if you're looking through the lens of a cheap camera. So we have to calculate, to take this distortion into consideration."

"Calculate?"

"Yes. But the amount of distortion is a known quantity. So we can make fairly precise calculations and corrections."

So they strap me down onto this table. And I've got my arms behind my head and they've got four guys, one at my feet, one at my head, one on each side, right and left. This is done downstairs, near the X-ray area. The room is set up with very bright lights and a film/videotape console. I was sweating from the lights. They have a little ring they put on your chest, where this biopsy needle fits into, and it has to go in at a certain specified angle.

Now you can imagine—they have these four doctors standing there. And this one doctor is saying to me, "John, I want you to remember that the one important thing is, when we get the biopsy needle *in,* and it's securely in *place*—when I say hold your *breath,* you hold your *breath.* OK? let's practice."

So I'm practicing. I take a deep breath and he says, "OK. Hold it." So I hold it. As long as I can. Then he says, "OK. Breathe." Well fine and dandy. I've got that down pretty good. There's only one problem about to come up. It's all well and good to take a deep breath *inward,* and hold it. Right? But just try and do the same thing while you're letting your breath *outward*! And stop at a point—and hold it! It's two different things. Which he didn't explain to me. That small goddamn little detail. That he might say hold your breath on an *exhale*!

So there's these four doctors standing all around me, and a technician, and a nurse from the cardiac care section, and one doctor is giving directions on the angle this biopsy needle has to go in. He's in the middle, and he's saying, "OK, fellas. How does it look from down there? Does it look like it's straight?" And the other guy says, "Yeah. Move it a *little* to the right." Then he goes to the guy on the right and asks, "Does it look like it's straight, to you?" "No. A little to the left."

Now you can just imagine how I'm feeling. Here you think these guys are all experts, and everything is super scientific. But they're playing this game by eyesight! And here I am, laying there, my life on the line, and I feel like this big overgrown guinea pig, and I'm saying to myself, Oh Jeez! I hope that guy in the middle, the team captain, I hope he didn't leave his glasses home today!

So then this middle doctor says, "OK, Mr. Hurley. We've got this thing lined up. OK. Now when I say hold your breath, you hold your breath. Just like we rehearsed it. All right?"

"Ready."

"*OK!*" So I take a deep breath. And I'm waiting for him to say hold it. And the seconds are ticking away. And I'm starting to let the air out, and it's just about all out, and I figure I'll have time to take another deep breath, when suddenly—I still can't believe this—suddenly he says "*HOLD IT!*" A command. And the needle goes into the middle of my lung! And I'm trying to hold my breath, and the spots are coming in front of my eyes, and my eyes are bulging out of their sockets, and I'm turning red and getting dizzy, and up there on the TV screen I see the needle in my chest sitting right inside my lung in living color, and my heart pumping away, and the spots are getting colored yellow now and flashing before my eyes, and I swear I'm gonna strangle or faint any second! And finally I hear it. "OK, John. You can relax. We've got it." *Bastards!*

After they pulled the needle out again, they played the videotape back that they were making. And just as the needle entered my chest, you could see it (in slow motion) just missing the aorta —by a *hair's* breadth! One of the doctors said, "Whoa! Close one!" Another one said, "You better believe it. Whoa!" They were all shaking their heads that the needle had missed me at all. Whoa!

"You're a lucky man, John."

"I know it, gentlemen. But thank you."

*"De nada."*

"Thank you very much."

Turned out that the spot was just a spot. Of unknown origin. It went away by itself. Was never heard from again.

Isn't that just *swell*? *Shmucks!*

Dot and Tom Costanza called up just after I was released again as an outpatient. They're friends from Sea-Land. He was one of the original wrecking crew. They drove up more than three hundred miles from Thousand Oaks, just to spend the weekend with us. He's an antique car buff. So naturally, we spent the day driving around looking for parts for his car. Costanza is a short and stocky Italian, with jet black hair, a real full, round face, and he's constantly cutting up, like a little Lou Costello.

That night we shot some pool in the rec room of the apartment. Then around ten-thirty that night, we got the itch. I felt it was still too early to go back to the apartment and call it a night. The girls had already turned in, saying they were bushed. So I said to Costanza, "Hey, Tommy. There's a bar I want to see, called "The Office." It's always intrigued me from the outside. But I've never seen the inside. How about you and me walking up to the corner and we'll go into this cocktail lounge, and we'll have a drink up there?"

Costanza says, "Sure thing, my man! Let's go!"

So we up and get to the door of this joint, step inside, and it turns out to be a very nice place. Very dark and plush. Red carpet. Walnut paneling. And we proceed to have a few and talk about old times in Puerto Rico. And one drink leads to another. And as the evening wears on, things start getting rougher and rougher in there. People started getting drunker and drunker. There were arguments all around us.

Costanza, who's maybe 5'6", turns to me and says, "John, what would happen if someone comes over and starts making trouble with us? I mean, how the hell am I gonna *protect* you? You're just out of the hospital, you're all stitched up with a new heart. Man, your chest is all wired up!"

I looked at him and said, "You save *your* ass, Costanza, and I'll save *mine*! Don't worry about it. Besides, I think I'm covered under Major Medical!"

Then the jukebox started playing, and this couple started a floor show. And she must have been a professional stripteaser. Or something close to it. Because they were dancing, and suddenly she starts putting on a show you wouldn't believe. That's why we didn't leave until three in the morning. She had no underwear on!

And she was smashed! She was amazing! After a while, her boyfriend was so embarrassed he didn't even want to dance with her any more. She was doing bumps and splits and everything else you can imagine, including sitting up on the tables and lifting her dress up to everybody, then jumping down onto the floor and doing whirls and grinds! With no panties on!

She was some gorgeous gal! This was some place! So as I say, one drink led to another. And I had to be up the next morning at 5:00 A.M. to be at the hospital at 6:00 for the outpatient tests.

Somehow, we got up on time. Two hours' sleep. And dragged ourselves over to the hospital. We were *wrecked*. But Costanza, being the real character that he is, he had the cure-all for the hangover he had. Takes a can of beer with him to the hospital! To nurse his head.

This was the first vacation he had taken away from his business for four years. And you talk about a mind. You've never met *anyone* with a memory like he has. *Photographic.* The real thing.

Always had it. Tommy Costanza could drive down a street that he's never been on before in his *lifetime,* and after that one time, he could tell you the name of the street he was on, the address of almost every store on *both* sides of the street (providing he had time to see them all), what each store's *name* was, and what they *sold*! Talk about a photographic memory. He has the mind of a *genius*!

*ANN* John's parents called often, asking how he was, and if I wanted them to come out and help. I said thanks, but I was managing.

I didn't let myself speculate about the future. At least I tried not to. But every once in a while I thought about what would happen if John didn't pull through. If a rejection set in. He'd already had one episode. That time they'd caught it. We were lucky. And it was an acute rejection, too. Also, the medication itself was extremely potent and risky.

That's when I was grateful that I had the younger children. I felt they would be something to live for. And that's what really kept me going. I had to keep going. I had to keep my wits about me no matter what was happening to John. Because I had the young ones at home. But I don't think I speculated as to how it would actually be—without John. Lonely, probably. I was frightened.

I'm frightened lots of times right now. In fact I'm frightened most of the time when I think about it. Of being by myself. Raising the children by myself. That's as far as I go. Then I just wake up.

Dr. Kroner said something to me a long time ago that really holds me together. "Ann, you've just got to realize that you and John are simply not going to retire together."

"I know that."

"Just be thankful for every day, every week, and every month you've had with him already. He's long outlived that heart he's got in that body. By all odds, he really should have been gone by now. And that's the bottom line."

I prayed a lot. Alone. At the hospital. I don't remember praying that much in my whole life. Constantly. Even when I'd be in his room. In fact, the rosary beads that I'd put away years back, they were with me constantly. The last thing I packed. Had them since I was a little girl. Prayed silently. Over him while he slept.

We couldn't go to the church at night. A week before we came out, they had found a woman decapitated in the chapel on the Stanford campus. Her head was cut off and she was completely sexually mutilated. Slit open with a razor from top to bottom. They thought it might be one of those fanatical religious groups or something. So the hospital put extra lights in the parking lots, and extra roving security guards and dogs, especially for when the nurses changed shifts.

# 21

## *Janice*

*ANN*  Janice just turned fifteen. She had to quit being a color guard in school because of working. Carried the American flag, and the different flags and guns of all nations. She carried the flag in front of the band last year. Wore a red, white, and blue uniform. With majorette boots. Last year the girls made their own uniforms. She twirled the flag.

Janice doesn't talk about boys with John or me. She doesn't say anything. I know she talks about them with her friends, because that's the only possible thing they could be giggling about so often. She tells me she'd like to go to college and study the science field. She'd love to be a veterinarian. But it's so many years of school. She loves animals and nature. She's had a lot of pets. Guinea pigs, dog, cat, turtles, fish. She works at the A&P after school. She's a cashier. She's saving up for her own car.

She was the only child for ten years, and then her whole life changed. Suddenly, she had a baby sister. Then everything piled up. Little John was born. And a month later big John had his heart attack. So nothing was the same for her ever again.

I've asked her many times if she resents her father, or her little sister and brother, and she says no, but I think that there has to be some kind of resentment. And I think it started to come out in California.

She began crying out for help—by acting up at Barbara's house. And from the sound of it, I felt that if we didn't bring her out to us at once, we might lose her for good. My sister Barbara did all she could to try and understand Janice. But with that, plus taking care of the two little ones, and her own three children as well—she was finally getting exasperated with Janice's behavior.

She called me to tell me she was having a serious problem with her. Janice and she had had a big fight. And Janice was being very belligerent and antisocial.

"That doesn't sound like Janice."

"I know it doesn't, Ann. That's what I'm trying to tell you. It isn't Janice the way we know her to be. She's changed. Really changed. And honest to God, we can't handle her any more."

I said to John, "I really think she's crying out for our help. And this acting up is the only way she knows how—because she's never been that kind of a disobedient girl. She's never given me any kind of trouble. You know that everybody's always liked her."

I think Janice was petrified. And this was her only way of showing how she felt.

When she got to California, I waited for her to come around and talk to me about the problems Bobbie and Ronnie had had with her. She didn't. So finally I came right out and asked her.

"So what happened with you and Bobbie and Ronnie?"

"What are you talking about?"

"I'm talking about back home. With Bobbie and Ronnie. They say you were turning everybody off. Freezing them out. Clamming up and refusing to talk to anyone."

"I did. And I'm not sorry. Because they don't need me. Just like you and Daddy . . . don't need me."

"But Janice, we love you very very much. And we do need you! We do! Where on earth would you ever get such an idea like that? Of course we need you!"

"No you don't! You don't have *any* time for me! Ever since Daddy got sick, you haven't had any time for me! It was always him first, or the kids."

"That's not true!"

"Yes it is. And you know it."

"Look Janice, your father has been a very sick man. You know that. So nothing that's been done has been done deliberately to you. But that doesn't explain what happened between you and Bobbie. What was the trouble? Why couldn't you all get along? Why did you fight all the time?"

"Because it wasn't my family. I missed you and Daddy and everything was getting on my nerves. Bobbie was yelling and screaming at me—all the time! And finally I yelled back! Then I went into my room and slammed the door real loud, and stayed there until the next morning."

I guess it's a frightening thing to a kid to be left with relatives while her parents go off to California for God knows what. I think she was scared shitless—and couldn't map out the whole thing. It happened so fast.

Janice felt that she wasn't wanted, wasn't loved, wasn't needed, and that we neglected her. She said she wasn't old enough to accept the responsibility—and that every time she tried to talk to us, we were preoccupied with something else. And it wasn't only John's medical attention. One day we might be drinking with our friends. The next day it was his friends at the airport. Or it was the little children, constantly.

"Janice, you must know that this was all unintentional."

"Whether you meant to or not, it was done, Mother."

"I realize that. Now. I really do."

"And I'm going to tell you something else. Something that I've given a lot of thought to."

"Yes?"

"I'm going to run away, Mother. I really mean it. I'm going to run away."

"You can't mean that."

"I do mean it, Mother. I've just about made up my mind."

"You can't be serious. You don't know what you're saying."

"I know very well what I'm saying. Look at me. I'm not crying. I'm very calm. And I've thought this out very, very carefully. I'm definitely leaving. And I'm not *ever* coming back again."

"Janice! Will you please stop talking like that? You're frightening me. We are a *family*! Don't look at me like that! That's right! I said a family! And any problems we may have, we can talk them out, and iron them out. Don't you ever forget that. We are a *family*. And we do love you. Very, very much. Maybe even more than you know!"

"I'm leaving. I don't know where I'm going to go. But I have to go away. Nobody cares about me! Even when you *left,* you didn't have any time for me! Plans were being made, everything was speeding up, everybody was running around—and I was *left out.* Of everything! I had *nobody* to talk to! And you said it would be different after his operation. But it still isn't really different. He still gets mad too fast. It's always been like that. It was worse before his operation. But it still really isn't any different. Maybe you understand, sometimes, but he never did. Daddy *never did*! He always yelled. Like with my grades. You would just say to bring them up. But he'd start yelling and stuff. I don't like it when he yells! He makes me so angry I could leave you all forever, and never see you again! I really mean it! I really do!"

"Janice, I—"

"Go away, Mother! Just go away and leave me alone! I'll do what I have to do! No matter what! I'm just gonna do what I have to do!"

"Janice—"

*"Leave me alone!"*

Then she went to sleep, sobbing to herself. Deep, heartfelt sobs. I wanted to go in to her and comfort her. But the mood she was in, I knew I could never get through to her.

This was pretty stiff stuff coming from a fifteen-year-old. All I could think of was how glad I was that John wasn't there at the time to hear this. He was at the clinic and hadn't come back yet. He'd be outraged.

I tried to weigh the possibilities. I wondered if Janice really meant it. Would she leave? And when? That night? The next day? And where would she go?

But then something told me that Janice wouldn't really carry out her threat. At least not yet. She was more concerned at this point with expressing the feelings that had been locked up inside her, building up to the breaking point for all these months. Or had it been years? That's what really worried me.

For the first time, I realized that we might not ever have properly understood what she was thinking and feeling and going through, as she had been growing up. I could hear her through her door, crying to herself. She still sounded like a baby to me. Really a little girl. But at the same time she was getting to be an adult. Growing up pretty quickly. And John and I hadn't really noticed, I guess. We had been so preoccupied with ourselves.

When John came home that afternoon, I fixed him lunch. And then I told him. And he said, "Ah . . . don't sweat it. She's fifteen. That's her age talking. You can't get upset over these little things."

"I don't think it's a little thing, John. I think it's very serious.

And could really mean something. That she could even *think* of leaving home!"

"Ah . . . every kid goes through that. Don't sweat it."

That night, she'd eat only in her room. I tried to talk to her more, and she would yes, yeah, and no me. That's all I could get out of her. The freeze was on. She got very distant. Treated us like complete strangers. Ignored us. Answered questions with yes and no but wouldn't hold a conversation with us.

After dinner, I went into her room, and had another talk with her. She never mentioned running away again. But this time she said I was waiting on John too much.

"I think you're out of control, Mother! You wait on him hand and foot! Like he was a baby or something. Why don't you cut his meat for him, too?"

"But Janice, your father is still a very sick man."

"You said he was OK."

"He is OK. But it's a matter of degree."

"I don't get it. Is he or isn't he OK?"

"Your father is OK for a man that has been through what he's been through. But it takes a long time to get back to full strength again. He's been through a serious operation."

"I still think you wait on him too much. How is he gonna get better if you don't let him do things for himself?"

"Janice. Let me explain something to you. There's something that I think you still don't understand about your father's condition."

"*What? What* don't I understand?"

"Janice . . . your father . . . just possibly . . . has five more years to live. Just possibly. Maybe seven . . . on the outside. We're talking about maybe five to seven more years to live. Do you understand what I'm telling you?"

"So? So what? That's a *long* time! How long does he *want* to live?"

And I was shocked. I thought to myself, My God, she really is a little brat.

A week later, it hit the fan.

Janice wanted something different for dinner than what we were having. She wanted pizza. I said OK. I went ahead and prepared it, and took it out of the oven and set it down in front of her, and it looked sensational. I was really proud of myself. It was sizzling like a mother. A masterpiece. And she looks down at it and says, "I'm not eating it. I don't want it any more." You know, typical teen-ager. She's going to spite me—and she isn't going to eat it.

"But Janice, you asked me for it. I made it for you, special."

"I don't care. I don't want it any more."

"Why not?"

"I'm not eating it. I'm not hungry any more."

"But I opened the package and made it just for you!"

"I don't care. It looks like a mess."

"A mess? It's gorgeous. Just look at it. It's delicious."

"I'm not eating it, Mother. I don't care what you say. I'm just not eating it. And you can't force me to, either. I'm just not going to have it. I don't want it any more."

"Janice, please. I went to a lot of trouble to make this for you—"

Well John is watching this, and all of a sudden he turns red. His eyes were fire. He started to scream. In fact, he got up from his chair and bellowed, "YOU'RE GONNA EAT IT—OR BY GOD YOU'RE GONNA BE *WEARING* IT! AROUND YOUR HEAD! YOU LITTLE BRAT!"

She just sat there, looking at him. "I don't want it. I'm not hungry."

"NOT HUNGRY? YOU'RE NOT HUNGRY? WELL THAT'S IT! THAT'S IT!" He turns to me. "That's it! I've had it! I've had it, goddamn it! We're being treated like garbage by this little brat! And by Christ I'm not taking it any longer! I mean it, Ann. I've taken all the guff I'm going to from this little brat! She sits in the same goddamn room with you, and you'd never even know she was there! Yes. No. Yes. No. What kind of crap is that? I mean, really! What the hell is going on here? What kind of behavior is this crap? Really! I'd like to know!"

"So would I, John. Something is really bothering this girl. She's really disturbed about something."

"Disturbed? Yeah, she's disturbed! Well I'm disturbed about this too!"

"Please, John. Don't yell at her. Let's try to work this out. If we just show a little patience and understanding, she'll calm down. She'll come around. I know she will."

"Well I'm not so sure. I'm really not so sure about that. How about it, Janice. Are you gonna eat that pizza that your mother made for you?"

"I'm not hungry any more. I don't want it!"

"YOU'RE GONNA EAT IT RIGHT HERE AND NOW OR I'M GONNA PUT YOU RIGHT THROUGH THAT WALL! AND IF YOU WANT TO, YOU CAN PACK YOUR GODDAMN BAGS AND GET THE HELL OUT OF THIS HOUSE! I'VE HEARD OF THESE RUNAWAYS, AND IF YOU HAVE ANY INTENTIONS ON THAT SCORE, PACK YOUR BAGS AND GET THE HELL OUT RIGHT NOW! WE DON'T NEED THIS KIND OF BEHAVIOR FROM A SPOILED LITTLE *BRAT*! GET OUT NOW! DAMMIT! WE DON'T NEED THIS KIND OF BULLSHIT! GO ON! *MOVE!*"

It was as blunt as that. Janice ran out of the room, in tears, and locked herself into her bedroom. I went after her, but she wouldn't open the door. I went back to John. He was steaming. He lit up a cigarette. The first one he'd had in months. He wasn't supposed to smoke. But I didn't dare say anything, the way he was feeling now.

Three hours passed. We tried to watch some television. But nothing really held our attention. Janice came out of her room and went into the kitchen. She poured herself a glass of milk and started back for her room (but through the living room, where we were). John got up, switched the TV off, and said, "Wait a minute, Janice. I want to talk to you. Sit down."

"What about?"

"Sit down, will you? Please?"

She sat down on the floor.

"Listen, Janice. I just want to say that . . . regardless of any mistakes that have been made in the past . . . and we did make some mistakes . . . we just want to reassure you. Your mother and I, we know it was a mistake in not sitting down with you more often, taking the time, explaining the situations . . . respecting your feelings more. Listen, Janice . . . we love you very much . . . regardless of how we might not express it. Even though we may not kiss and hug you all the time . . . we still love you. I know that all of this has been hard on you, that we saddled you with too much responsibilities and things back home . . . like watching the babies all the time, and things like that, and not taking the time to explain everything to you. We realize that now. And we realize that we might have taken advantage of you back home, by using you as a babysitter too often, because every opportunity we had to get out and get away from the babies, I guess we did. I realize that now. So I *promise* you, when we get home, things'll change. Things are going to be different. Just let us know that you have some prearranged party you're going to, or plans for a date, and we'll pay a babysitter, rather than make you stay home with the kids. How's that? OK?"

"OK."

"OK. Then let's kiss and make up and all be friends again. Right?"

"Right, Dad."

The night ended very quietly. He cried. I cried. Janice apologized to him for acting up, and kissed him. She's exactly like he is. They know each other perfectly. She reassured John that she loved him. Always did and always will.

Looking back on it now, I can honestly say and admit to myself that I failed her. I think . . . I *hope* I've won her back. I was petrified of losing her. I felt that if we didn't get through to her pretty soon, we were going to lose her for life. If she's asking for help at fifteen, there's a problem.

But, despite what he had said to her, I honestly believe that John, deep down, refused to believe that she had a deep-rooted problem. John doesn't like to make mistakes and doesn't like to admit them. So he put it on babysitting terms, and like that.

I really think that was the tip of the iceberg as far as Janice was concerned.

**JOHN**  I don't readily admit mistakes. As far as work is concerned, I can't ever remember doing anything that really screwed things up, that was really a mistake.

When I was a kid and made a mistake, my mother or father would probably smack me in the head. But they really thought the sun shined out of my ass.

As far as Janice is concerned, I'm very quick tempered. When she first came out to California, she wasn't easy to get along with. She was rebellious. She had almost a complete personality change from the time we left. She was distant. Sullen. Introverted. One minute she'd be up, the next minute depressed. Wouldn't talk.

I'm not tolerant. I always look for respect. I didn't feel I was getting respect. In a sense I think that was part of the problem. I don't believe in having debates with children.

But looking back, we didn't take the time with Janice to show her she was loved. To explain things to her. To help her understand. We expected too much of her. All she wanted was to know she was loved. This was the basis of the blowup with me. She felt that she could not sit down and talk a situation out with me.

I sat her down and told her, "Look Janice, maybe we don't *show* you—I have a different way of expressing myself than your mother has—but we love you *very much.*"

Ann had a hangup, and wanted Janice to go to a psychologist. But I don't believe in psychologists. That's my own personal belief. I think if you have something to go talk to someone about, and you wanna sit down and talk to someone who is gonna be compassionate and listen to you and possibly offer some comfort to you, then you should go to someone who is a religious person, who has a theological background. But I don't believe in psychologists. Or psychiatrists.

It's hard being a teen-ager. But by the time Janice turns eighteen, it'll be different. Because fifteen to seventeen is a terrible age anyway.

# 22

## Rest and Relaxation

*JOHN* Ann and I had our first sex together.

It was six weeks after I was discharged as an outpatient. February '75. I had been told by a doctor that there were no sex restrictions whatsoever.

"Go to it, champ. More power to you. It's healthy for you. And as a matter of fact, your heart is six years younger than you are!"

I wasn't afraid that the excitement and exertion would affect me. They say when you worry about it, it's with a stranger. Not when you're with your wife!

Only kidding, Ann!

As an outpatient, we had a lot of time in between. And there would be days when it would be raining and you wouldn't go out, so we'd stay home, puttering around.

We discovered this leather-working place in Palo Alto, run by a couple of young college kids. California is very big on leather crafts, so we developed hobbies, making pocketbooks, stamping leather, and stuff like that.

I got started with leather from my physical therapy at the hospital. They asked me what I'd like to try, and I thought of Janice mentioning she saw a nifty pair of moccasins she wanted, made out of leather. So I made her a pair. And she really liked them. It was easy. The hospital had all the tools and knives and different dies and stamps.

Later on we bought our own tools and supplies, and I made a pocketbook for Ann's sister Barbara, and little leather belts for Joanie and little John. I loved working with leather.

But not as much as visiting the wineries. We visited quite a few of them. Paul Masson, Brookside, Christian Brothers. They were great. The best part was the sampling part. After they took you on the tour and showed you how the wine is fermented and stored, bottled and corked, they gave you samples of all the wines they made. And they had a retail shop where they sold the wine that you liked.

We'd be smashed after going through the line! They had so many samples! Like Paul Masson's—they must've had fifty different kinds, and you could sample all of them if you wanted to. There's a sampling room. It's like a barroom, really. You can sit at tables and they'd come around with the different kinds of wine. They even had a *chocolate* wine!

I think this is where Ann got to enjoy wine.

Sometimes we went back a number of times. Brookside was only two and a half blocks from where we lived. So we paid *them* a few visits! It's open all the time. You'd just stop in and sample wine. We always bought some wine, though. My favorite was what they call Gamay Beaujolais. A red wine, similar to a burgundy.

It was very quiet when Janice left to go back home. She had

always been bugging us with "Let's go play miniature golf." Or "Let's go shopping."

But after she left, it was sort of quiet. I felt kind of lonely, I guess.

She had to go back to school. She'd been out a month and had to be back for the start of the second semester. At the airport, Ann and I were upset that she was leaving. But we knew it would only be a matter of weeks until we went home ourselves.

Janice held us tightly and then got on the plane.

One Thursday, after I was finished at the clinic, Ann and I went to the cafeteria to get some lunch. And we bumped into the psychologist again, Sylvia. She asked us how we were getting along and if there were any problems adjusting to the changes in our lives. We got to talking over coffee.

When I took my twelve o'clock medications, Sylvia asked me if I'd had any side effects from them.

"There *are* side effects, from the Prednisone. Ann would be making the beds, and two or three mornings in a row she found quite a bit of my hair on the pillows and sheets. At first she didn't say anything to me, but then she finally called me in to show me all the hair that was on the pillow. I said, 'My God, I'm losing my hair!' I ran to the mirror and started looking. "It don't feel any thinner!' I kept feeling my head. Then I took a shower and watched even closer to see if it was clogging up the drain. It was. So we told the doctors. They said that once they start reducing the dosage, it'll grow back, thicker. But that wasn't the worst of the problems. Another side effect was a *rash*—that showed up on my *balls.*"

"John!" Ann says.

"Maybe I oughta whisper this, huh? The doctors couldn't do a thing for it. Drove me up the wall with itching! So one day, Ann got a tremendous idea. She throws away this tube of useless gook the doctors gave me, and she goes out to the local drugstore, and comes home with this A&D ointment that they use for baby diaper rash. And by gosh it did the trick! I'm tellin' ya, the doctors were *amazed.* First, she spread the stuff all over my balls. Then she covered them with gauze. And next, a layer of *Saran wrap,* so it wouldn't stick to my sensitive skin. Then she topped everything off with her *hair drier. Heat* treatments! I tell you, this woman is *remarkable!*"

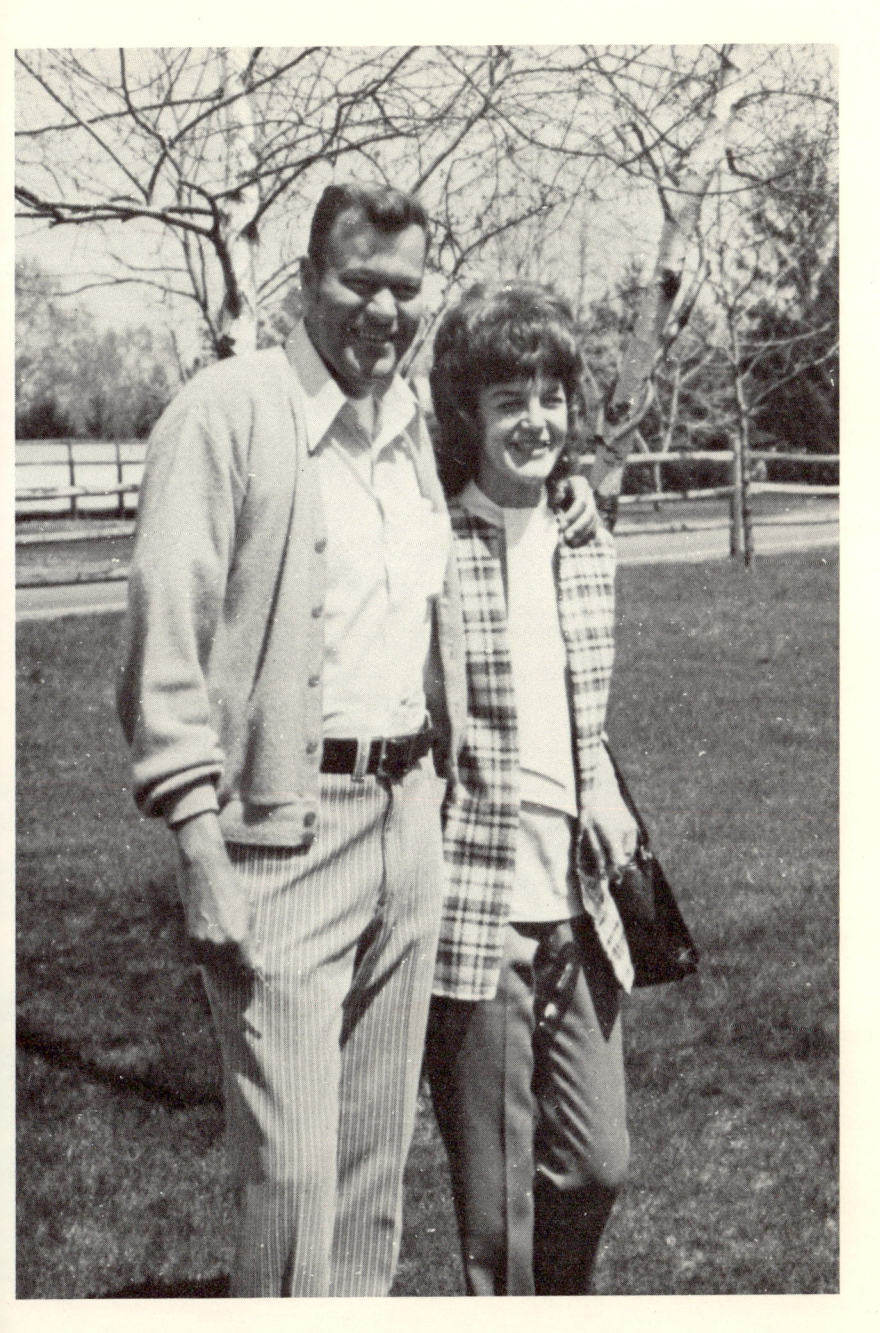

Right after John's promotion

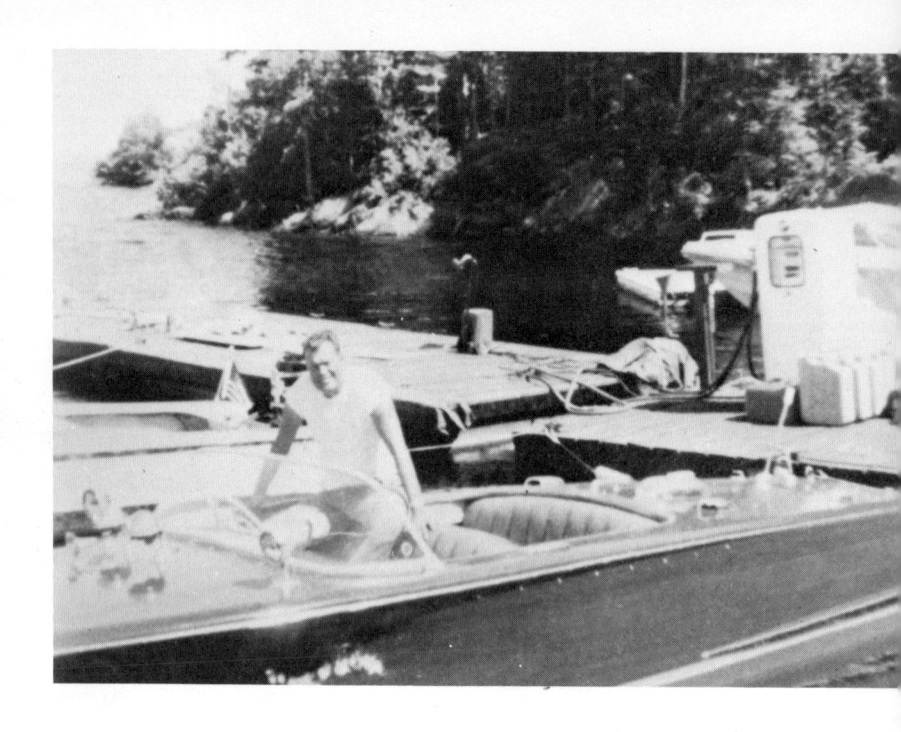

*Above* A gentleman of leisure
*Right* Going out for the evening
*Far right, below* Caribbean cruise

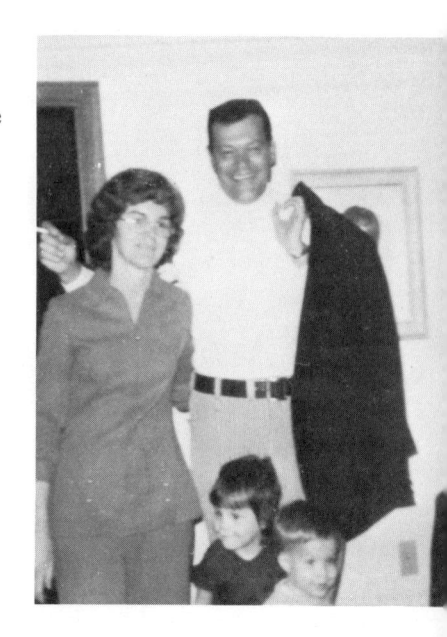

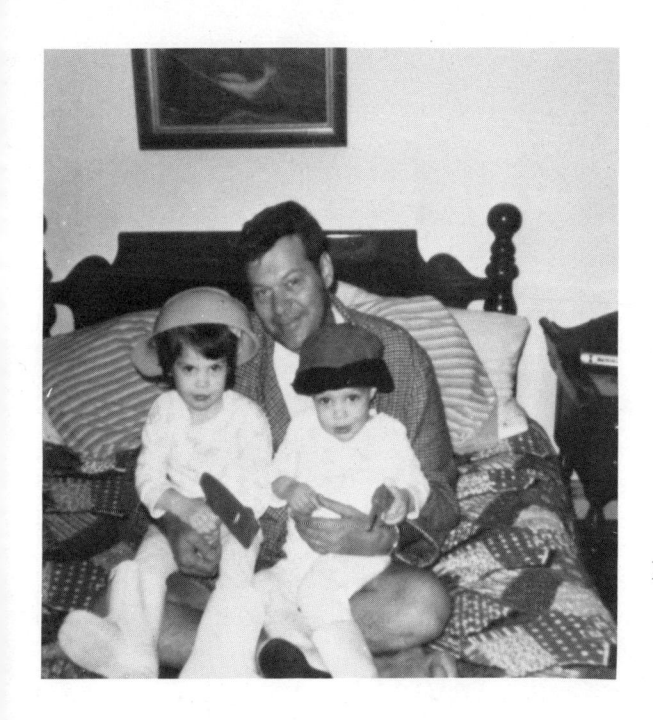

In retirement

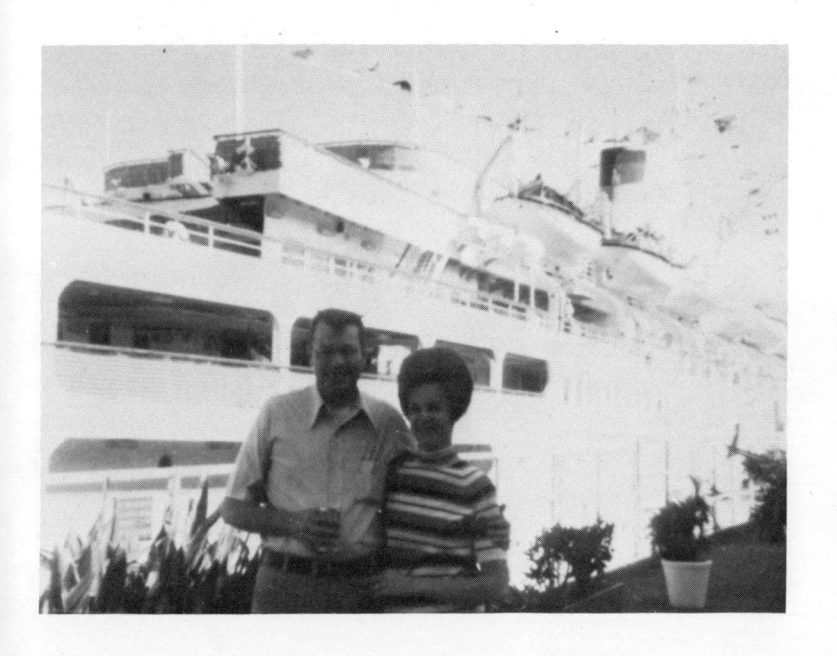

DEAR MR HURLEY

We were en the store I saw a big sign It was bout you but I dedent under stand Mom sed that ws caus I ws litle so she splaynd two me I stil Dont under sand I no wit out many you wil dy Plese dont dy I savd all my penys for you and I pray for you evry nite My daddy dy you must Be somebodys daddy so dont dy caus they wil be sad

Love
BJ

A letter from B.J.

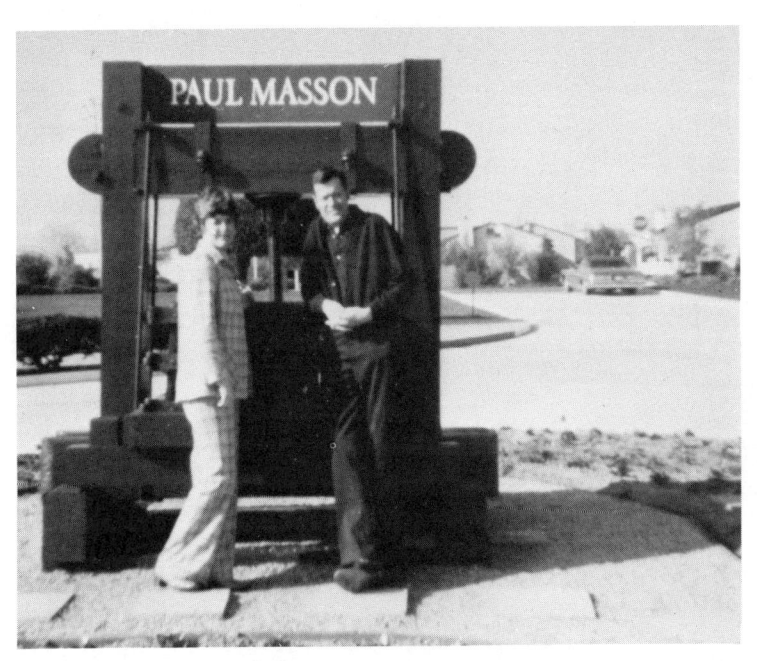

Visiting the wineries in California

John and Janice, California

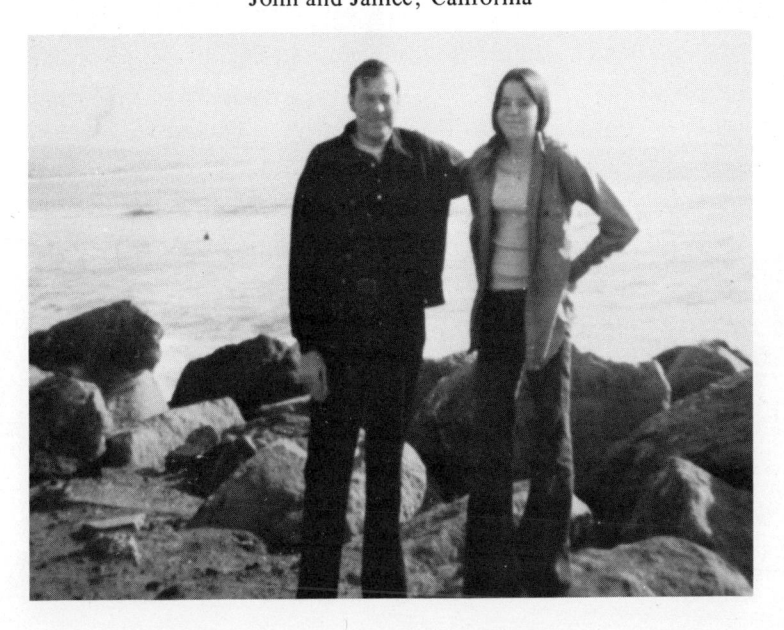

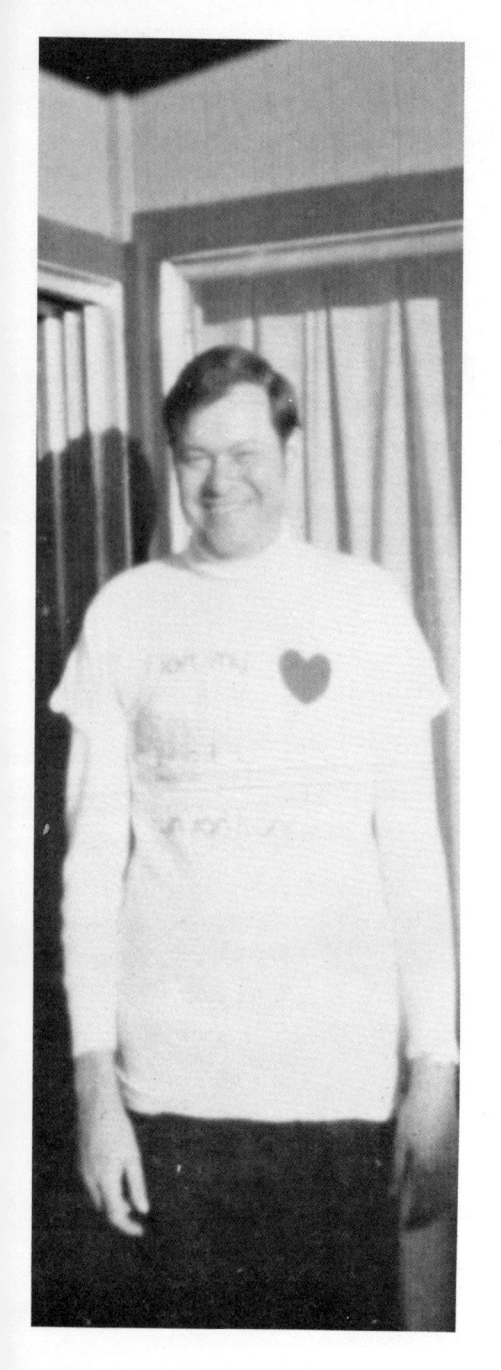

*Left* John with new heart

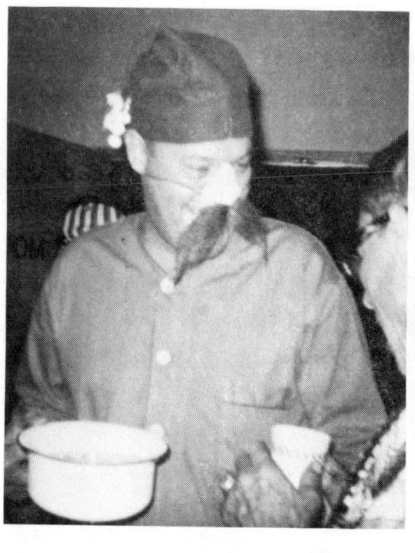

Feeling stronger every day

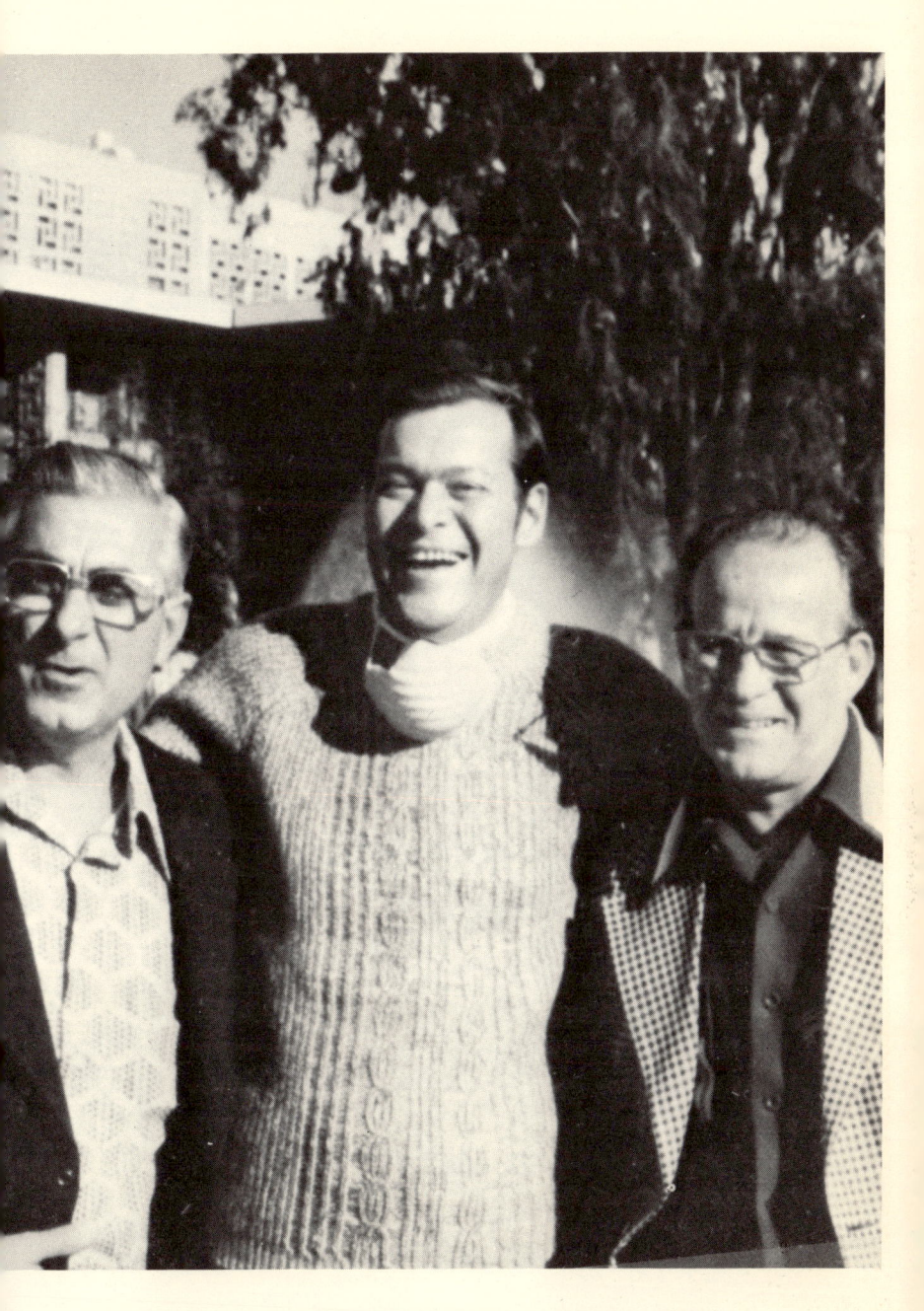

Released as an outpatient with Fred Kelly and Lincoln Blakely

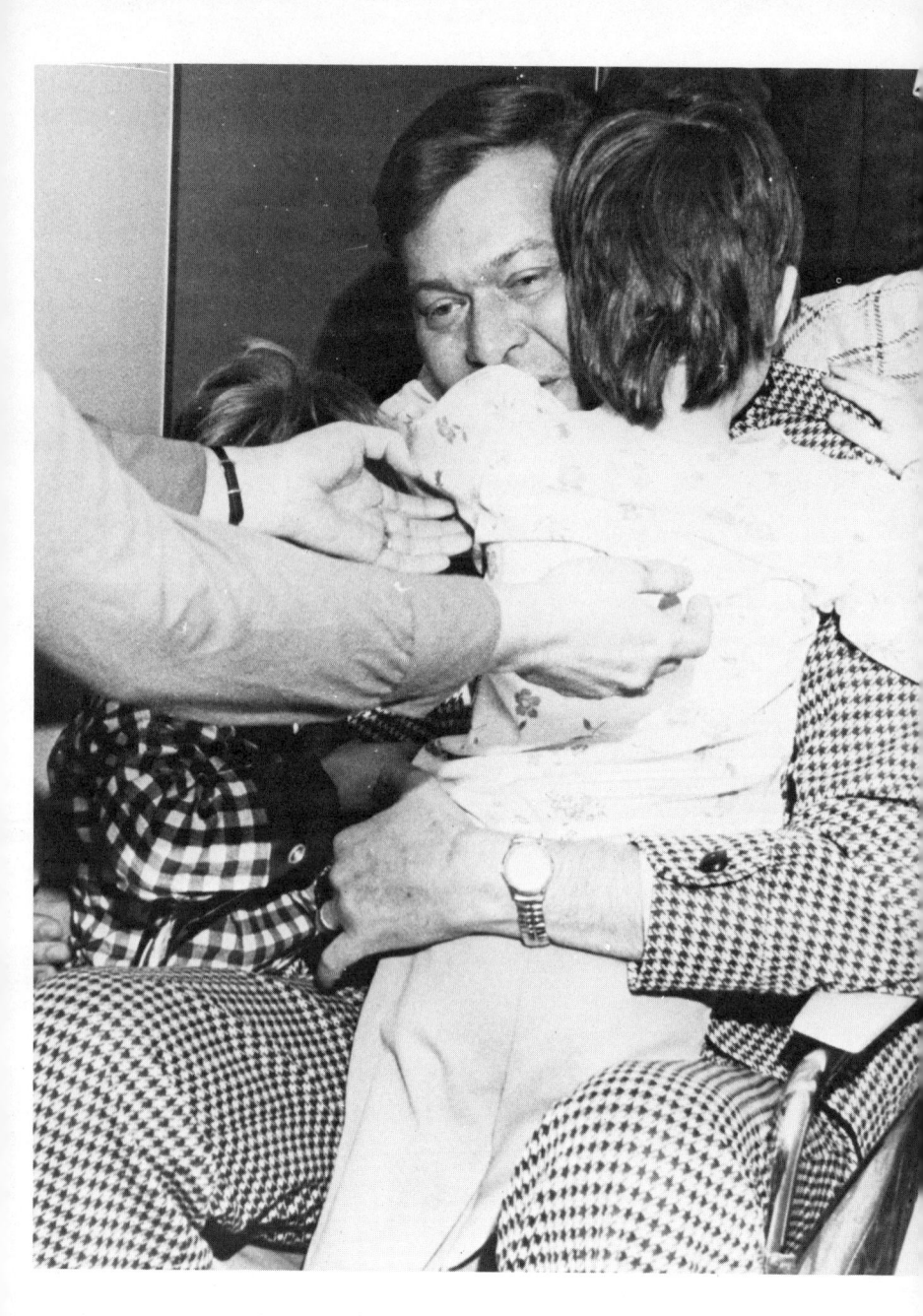

Home

# THREE

## A TRUCE WITH TIME

## 23

## *Return Ticket*

***JOHN*** I told my doctors I wanted to go home for my son's birthday, because it might be the last birthday I'd ever spend with him. They originally told me I'd have to be out there for as long as six months, as candidate, patient, and outpatient. But I heard that one of the transplants got out of there in less than six. So when I heard that, I was bound and determined to leave in less time.

I told 'em, "I don't care how you people work it out, but I'm leaving come St. Patrick's Day to be home with my boy on his birthday."

They were amazed at my progress. I was one of the earliest transplants to be released from both the hospital and from outpatient status. Three months and change. Released February 26th. I really think it was my mental attitude. I felt optimistic about my chances and got stronger every day. Ann had a lot to do with this.

Dr. Shumway is a hell of a man. A miracle man. Extremely

dedicated. And as kind and considerate and as decent a human being as you'll ever find. Whenever I saw him in the hall, he'd walk over, shake my hand, and we'd chat for a few minutes. He's not a power freak at all. Frankly, I'd never heard of the man before we went out for the transplant. Never. I heard of Barnard and DeBakey. But this man never seeks publicity or limelight. He has a way about him that's just so down to earth. I feel I've made a friend for life.

Before we left, we went to his office and spoke to him. I told him, "Doctor Shumway, you've given me the rarest gift in the world. I've heard of people receiving rare things, but I think you have given me one of the rarest things that a person can possibly receive. The gift of life. Talk of Limited Editions! This is really the way I feel, Doc."

He was very self-effacing. "It's not me, John. It's our whole surgical team, and the entire medical staff here at the hospital. Everyone working together here makes it all possible."

We shook hands, and I thanked him again. Then he escorted us to the front entrance of the building. We said our good-byes. He wished Ann and me the very best of luck and told us that if ever there was a problem, all we had to do was call. We thanked him again, and then I handed him a little gift we bought for him. A little hand-carved miniature statue of a surgeon, with a *saw* in one hand, and a scalpel in the other. And a stethoscope around his neck. He smiled when he saw it.

We flew home Thursday, February 27, 1975. A clinic day.

Phil Mazzucca, one of our neighbors, arranged for one of those real long limousines to pick us up at Newark Airport. I thought it was terrific! It was a freezing cold night, but it had a bar in the back. Janice, Joanie, and John Jr. were in the back with us. I had a couple of drinks coming home, being chauffeured, and it was a very nice feeling. The kids were very happy to see us. And it was likewise with us.

We drove up to the house, went inside, and a lot of our friends, neighbors, and relatives were waiting for us. They had arranged a buffet. Everyone was eating and drinking and having a good time. Jerry and Georgia Wood, and Shirley and Jules Berkowitz were there. And so were Jim and Jean Clark, Ann's parents, Patsy and Dennis McKenna, Barbara and Ronnie, Norene and Berndt, Lee and Lennie Tallo, Jan and Rich Traeger, Marie and Phil Mazzucca, the Gonzalezes, Walter and Mary Dignan, Donna and Steve Maroon, Jimmy and Miriam Knobloch, and all their kids shouting, "Uncle John is home! Uncle John is home!" And a couple of reporters from the local papers.

I felt tremendous. Just to be home. It was a terrific feeling of freedom. People were stopping in and saying hello all night long. It was exhausting but still felt good to me. I was just sitting in the rocking chair in the living room, presiding over the proceedings like a very thin Henry the Eighth!

I even had a few gifts to hand out. Before we flew home, I said, "You know, Ann? There's one thing I want to do. I want to buy something for each member of the family." So I went out and bought specially registered Wells Fargo belt buckles for each one of them. Bought ten of 'em. They're collector's items. Limited Editions on 'em. Registered with a serial number and everything. And on the back is inscribed their name, and the date of my heart transplant. November 16, 1974. As a remembrance. A keepsake.

After it was over and everyone went home, I couldn't get out of my rocking chair. I couldn't move my back. But it was still great. You can't appreciate something like that unless you've been away for a long time. It's sort of like returning home from a war after being a prisoner for ten years. A homecoming.

I was exhausted. I looked around the living room. It was a

wreck. Empty glasses, ashtrays filled to the brim, plates all over, empty booze bottles. But it was home. I looked at the pictures of the family over on the hutch. My parents. The kids. God it was good to be here!

Gretchen, my hunting dog, came over and sat down next to me. She had been hanging back all evening, just checking me out. But now she was nuzzling against my feet.

"That's a good dog, Gretchen! You old pal o' mine! How are ya?"

I petted her, and she let out a few good barks.

"That's a good girl. That's a good girl. That's a good girl! That's my girl! That's my good girl!"

A couple of weeks later, who shows up on our doorstep but Reuben Barclay! Our friend from Sea-Land's Oakland, California, office. And Reuben is bearing a gift. He hands me an envelope. He's got this big Cheshire cat grin on his face. I open it. There's a letter inside.

March 11, 1975

Dear Mr. Hurley,

The enclosed check comes to you from the employees and friends of Sea-Land in California, along with our collective best wishes that you will continue to receive His blessings.

Thank you for letting us participate in—and thus perhaps become at least a small part of—this modern miracle.

We hope your experience can be a source of encouragement and inspiration to others faced with a similar situation.

    Very truly yours,
    SEA-LAND SERVICE, Inc.
    Reuben A. Barclay, for
    all Sea-Land Employees

I almost dropped my drawers.

I knew that Reuben and Fred Kelly and Mike Ladner had been working through the company to help us out. There was a blood donation program. And they had planned an in-company raffle. And I knew about a cocktail party they were going to have, with prizes being donated. The money from the ticket sales was going to be forwarded to us, to defray some of our expenses. But for the moment, I had completely forgotten about it.

Ann and I felt badly that we were unable to attend the cocktail party, but it was scheduled for two weeks after I was due to be released from the hospital. So I wrote a letter to thank everyone for their help. The employees of Sea-Land, longshoremen, truck drivers, customers, people who owned liquor stores, you name it, everyone who donated the prizes for the raffle.

The grand prizes were a weekend at Lake Tahoe for two, and use of a completely furnished three-bedroom luxury apartment with maid service; and a trip to the Island of Hawaii for a week, for two.

Other prizes were a Marriott Inn weekend for two, including champagne and Marriott money; two nights for two on the *Queen Mary,* deluxe; a cruise for two to Catalina Island; various tickets for the LA Dodgers, Kings, and Lakers, Warriors, Seals, and Oakland A's; a Black & Decker garage vacuum cleaner; a full-course Japanese dinner for six people, prepared and served in your own home by kimono-clad hostesses, courtesy of Yonemoto and Angeli; $75.00 in cash, donated by the members of the John Swett High School Sugar City Super Band, from Crockett, California; a Voit bowling ball, donated by Albany Bowl; a macrame pot holder (believe it or not), made by Debby Pericola; and a one-hour musical concert held under your window, given by one of the local bands!

This is only the smallest sampling of what those people did for us. I can't remember all of it!

So when the night of the cocktail party came, Reuben read my letter to everyone who was there. And my letter quoted another letter, a letter from "BJ," one of the anonymous contributors to the Fund. And perhaps the most memorable contributor of all.

Dear Friends,

I am sorry that we cannot be with you tonight, and hope that the evening will be as memorable for you as it is for us.

In these uncertain times, it is most gratifying that all of you would take the time to do as much as you have, for one insignificant, unimportant, and largely unknown person like me.

We have all heard about people receiving fabulous gifts of rare and valuable First Editions. I can assure you that I have received from all of the wonderful people in California the rarest gift of all—in your repeated kindnesses. The letters, cards, best wishes, prayers, and the blood donations—not to mention your practical generosity shown by your activity this evening. All of these things have provided great inspiration during my operation and recuperation.

It is difficult to find the proper words to express our feelings, so please allow me to quote from a letter I received, written by a young child who had seen a John Hurley Fund poster displayed in a store by our friends in New Jersey. He was very young indeed. We do not know his identity. He preferred to remain anonymous. But the letter—a letter from "BJ," for that's how he signed it—said: "Dear Mr. Hurley. We were at the store. I saw a big sign. It was about you but I didn't understand. Mom said that was because I was little so she explained me. I still don't understand. I know without money you will die. I saved all my pennies for you and I pray for you every night. My daddy died. You must be somebody's daddy so don't die because they will be sad. Love, BJ."

Enclosed with the letter was a one-dollar bill.

Just let me say that as a father of small children, this touched me very deeply. How grateful I am that I now have the precious gift of more time to try to guide my own children to help them become the same type of compassionate and thoughtful adults you have proved to be.

                Sincerely,
          John and Ann Hurley and family

March 17th. St. Patrick's Day rolled around. John Jr.'s birthday.

We had a small party in the kitchen. Ann bought a huge ice cream cake with four candles on it. We kept it hidden from the little ones as a surprise. And when the time came, I put on a big white chef's hat and brought the cake to the table. Little John was tickled by it. He really liked it. He made a silent wish, then blew out the candles. Everybody clapped their hands and said, "Yaaaay!"

While we were singing "Happy birthday to you, happy birthday to you," Ann and I looked at each other. We both had tears in our eyes. "Happy birthday, dear John, happy birthday to *you*!"

I had made it home for his birthday.

I was home for good.

# 24

## Recovery at Home

*ANN*  At six in the morning, the alarm goes off. I get up. Wake John up. And the little ones are usually right up behind me. They don't give me five minutes. The baby wants his breakfast immediately. To keep him quiet I give him a bowl of corn flakes or Cap'n Crunch. A few minutes later, John comes up and he has his tea, his juice, and his medicine. Joan is starting her breakfast also. After she's made sure her daddy has had all his pills. She's his nurse. She's a pancake eater. Then little John has his second breakfast. Pancakes also. With maple syrup. Now I go down and wake up Janice. Which is impossible. But I try. Then I make lunches for the kids to take to school, peanut butter sandwiches on white bread, without the crusts, juice in a thermos, a Yodel, and fruit. By this time, the radio is on and John is shaving to it.

Then I blow my cool. Every morning. Because I'm not a morning person. I start yelling at the kids. Which does no good whatsoever. They're tuned out and far more interested in throwing pancakes than listening to their mother. Janice usually grabs a piece of toast and a swig of juice as she's running out the door to the school bus. She goes to Lenape Valley High School. Joanie marches out next, to Faith Christian School. Little John doesn't go to school yet, so he stays with me.

Then usually I'm straightening up the house, making beds, raking leaves, mowing the lawn. And the routine starts over again when the kids come home from school. Preparing for dinner, straightening the house, weeding, sweeping, driving Janice to work, shopping, doing the laundry at night. Because really . . . John . . . most of the things around the house he's not capable for any more. He's not supposed to mow a lawn. He can't go grocery shopping because he tires too fast. And he can't be lifting the heavy bundles. Not yet, anyway. So there are times when I can honestly say I could chuck the whole thing. I feel that after all we've been through, we haven't come any further. Except that John's still alive.

That's the way I feel. I can't help it. Nothing's been taken off my shoulders. Everything's been left to me. I don't like constantly screaming at the kids. I hate to. But then I go outside and see the leaves piling up, the lawn getting to be a mess, the car needing a wash, the dog needing to be fed, the bills having to be paid—just a lot of little things—and it seems to be too much on me lately. I said to John the other day, "If I don't come home one of these days, don't be surprised. I'm gonna leave you. You'll see. I'm gonna do it."

I keep blaming him. But then I realize it's not his fault. The pressures. None of this is his fault. I have to stop and remind myself. Because I really thought that things were gonna be a lot different after his operation. I thought he'd be entirely back to his old self again. *I was dead wrong.*

When we got back from Stanford, the first thing I did was to make sure he didn't have to cope with anything. It was always quiet in the house. Like a tomb. I'd make sure the kids got to bed early. I never let them play in our bedroom or go near him. I took them for walks as often as possible. Janice never had company. Teen-agers came over once or twice and didn't come back again, because they had to be so quiet.

Everybody catered to him. Treated him with kid gloves. So without realizing it, he started dodging his responsibilities again. By staying in his room like a hermit. For three meals a day. And I was being stupid enough—an ass, in plain English—to wait on him. Just like it was when he had his heart attack years before. I would bring his breakfast down to him. Then later in the day, he'd have a friend over and sit with him in the kitchen, having a couple of drinks—and as soon as his friend left, he would retire to his bedroom downstairs.

And that was His Lordship's little domain. Nobody could enter it. The kids could not go in to see him. He didn't want to be bothered. Every once in a while he would say, "Hello. How are you?" Then, "Get out. You're annoying me." I think he was getting so used to this little enclosure, and taking care of himself, that if somebody *sneezed,* they weren't allowed near him for the next two days. He became positively a hypochondriac. Finally I had to say, "You've got to live with them, John. Or you've got to move out to a hotel. When they're sick, I can't just put them out in the yard!"

There were a lot of these little confrontations. The anger and resentments were just building up inside of me daily. And then one day I hit bottom and saw red.

A friend of his had been here and they had had quite a few drinks together, in the kitchen. Then the friend left. John turns to me and points to the table where all the empties were and says, "Clean this up for me, willya Ann?" Then, the Master retired downstairs to his quarters.

I went after him, furious. "John, you come right back up here and clean this table up yourself. You're not crippled!"

And he yells up, "Nah. I'm tired. And my back is bothering me. You do it, willya kid?"

I think that suddenly—at that moment—the pressures got to be too much on me. I was taking more tranquilizers than I should. I started shouting at him. "What the hell is going *on* with you, John? When someone's here with you, you're smart as a whip, and joyful and happy. And you're drinking like a fish! But as soon as they leave, it's the *pits*! What is it? I'm *trying* to understand! Is it the children you resent? Is it me? Is it the house? I just can't deal with this crap any more! You're like a bloody hermit! I just can't understand it!"

And he couldn't either. But it was his way of avoiding any little domestic frictions—like at the dinner table. You know what a dinner table can be like, with young children. One spills milk, or they're giggling all the time. Another is throwing vegetables. As soon as he came to the table, he'd tell the children, "If you don't behave, I'm not eating with you any more." This is on the rare occasion that he *did* come to the dinner table.

I said, "Who the hell are you? Jesus Christ or something? Or are you Hitler? Life is very easy if you're just gonna sit alone by the boob tube or with a book, and someone is going to cater to your every whim! Well goddamn it, John, I'm not going to live on any fucking tranquilizers for the rest of my life! If you don't move out of that fucking bedroom, and get off your goddamn lazy ass, and assume some responsibilities in this goddamn fucking house—I'm gonna *kick you the hell out*!"

He was dumbfounded.

"When things are going wrong and the kids are screaming, and I'm having problems, there isn't anybody here to help *me* with them! I've taken the whole responsibility for *four fucking years* while you were so sick, and I couldn't tell you anything, and I had to hush the children. But now that you have a good new heart, you *still* don't accept any responsibilities! So what the hell's going on here? I think I'm being *fucked over*! Well—*shit on this!*"

"Ann, I—."

"I've had it! I'm being treated like a *fucking slave!*"

**JOHN** Which I accept. She was right. But Ann is overlooking something. Even if I *weren't* home all day, and was still out working, she'd *still* have to go through what she goes through from six in the morning till late in the day! Minus the maid service, of course.

But there's another thing, also. I don't know quite how to put this. But since the transplant—I don't *want to get too close to the kids*. That's right. It's a conscious decision. Because I know I only have a limited time left. When I do pass away, I think it's gonna have a profound psychological effect on the kids, if I get too close to them now. I think I'm doing them a favor—by keeping my distance. I've *never* been the type of a father that has been extremely close to the children. Never. I've always felt that it's my responsibility as the head of the household to provide the financial means of this family's existence. And Ann's responsibility is to provide the upbringing for those children. Period. Maybe that's chauvinistic. But that's the fact of it.

Since the transplant, I've been trying to set up a means, so that, if I were to pass away, Ann can continue to have the same life-style—only without me. I'm trying to provide a means of an education for Janice. So she is set and on her way to going to college. I don't have to be closely attached to Janice to do this. I can do this while being somewhat remote from her. I can. Hopefully I'll be around another year. At least I look forward to it. But once I pass away, the disability payments from work cease right there. Ann is left with life insurance. She's entitled to something nominal on Social Security. And that's what she's left with. That's *it*. Zip money. The insurance doesn't go far for long when you've got three children to feed, clothe, and educate. So believe me, it's on my *mind*. God! How I wish I could make money for my family. Even a little money. But I just can't. So *far*.

Finally, I avoided family responsibilities for another reason. My back. I really had a pain in my back. It was severe like anything. I really think Ann's forgotten this. This was the end of March. I was developing—without anybody realizing it—a severe infection. Creeping up on me. I couldn't move, it hurt so much. Once I lay down, I couldn't get up again. The pain was excruciating. Unbearable. It once took *three hours,* with Ann and my brother-in-law helping, to just get me out of bed.

ANN   It's true. You couldn't move him. Every inch of him, every little thing we touched on him he screamed afterwards, because of the pain. We got him to the edge of the bed and that was no good. So we had to bring him all the way back. Inch by inch. And then start all over again. It was excruciating for him. You had to be here to see it and believe it. It took three hours! My brother Jimmy finally *lifted the mattress,* physically, and we got John out of bed and into a wheelchair. We were exhausted.

I got John a drink and we talked for a little while.

Later, I went down to the doctor and told him what happened, and he suggested a hospital bed. We ordered it, and the next day the volunteer squad from the Roxbury Township brought it up to us.

Two nights later, John started feeling nauseous. It was real bad. I called Dr. Kroner's office, and his associate came right over. He checked John and said, "I'm afraid it's appendix. We'll have to go to the hospital." Then he called Dr. Kroner in New

York, where he was attending a seminar, explained the problem, and Dr. Kroner said, "I'll meet you at the hospital."

The ambulance gets here, siren wailing, the attendants rush in, and John tells them to hold everything—until he finishes his cigarette and martini!

The ambulance driver says, "What the hell's going on here? You're supposed to be a sick man."

And John says, "I'm not leaving until I finish my martini and my cigarette. That's not so hard to understand, is it?"

And everybody's standing around watching him! By now there were at least six people, including the chief of police, his deputies, and the ambulance crew!

John stalled for at least *eight more minutes*; then he took one last drag, one last sip, put the cigarette out in the ashtray like he was Adolphe Menjou, and turned to the ambulance attendants. "Very well, gentlemen. I'm yours."

They carried him up the stairs and out to the ambulance.


*JOHN* They rushed me down to Dover General. Dr. Dellessio took out my appendix. And then he found the demon that had tormented me all these months. It was the size of my hand, and growing on the inner lining of my muscles. My temperature was way up. Dangerously high. I'd been ripe for an infection because of the immunosuppressive drug therapy I'd been taking. They gave me massive antibiotics. They took hold. I started getting better.

I wanted to get out of the hospital no later than opening day of trout-fishing season. I was pushing the doctors. And they cooperated. I think they had had enough of me. They let me out on a Friday, and the next day, the season began.

But I couldn't go fishing yet because I was really bushed. Whacked out. My back was still sore and I could hardly walk.

## Recovery at Home

I was in a wheelchair again. The guys who I belong to this fishing club with, they knew that I wanted so badly to get out of the hospital to go fishing—and they knew I *couldn't* go fishing—so they set something up for me.

Trout season opens at eight in the morning, so what they did is, they all got together at six in the morning down at the Mountainside Diner and they all had breakfast. Then they all got in their boats, went out on the lake, and went fishing. So, they're drinking beer and what have you, and after they went fishing, they went over to the Tamarack, and they were drinking some more. And that's where they all decided they were gonna come up to my hospital room with this tremendous ice-chest cooler—this thing was 5 feet long and 3 feet wide, stocked with two dozen trout in it, and they were gonna bring along a fishing pole! *So I could go fishing in my room!*

The guys were half smashed, and these guys don't give a rat's ass for anyone or anything. And I mean that only in the very best sense. And they were gonna bring this huge Styrofoam cooler into the hospital! Sure, they have guards down there, but believe me, they couldn't have stopped those guys. Nothing could have. They would have picked up the guards and carried them bodily along with them. Straight into my room! But—unbeknownst to them—I had gone home the night before! So whattaya think they did?

As soon as they found out I'd been discharged, they came marching right up to the house, wheeled me straight out of the bedroom—before I could say a word—and right there in the middle of the backyard, they planted me and this tremendous cooler thing with two dozen shining little beauties in it! Then they stuck the fishing pole in my hand—and I just sat back in my wheelchair and cast into the cooler to get my fish! Some of them were 20 inches long!

Little John helped his old man. He hooked 'em, and I reeled

'em in. Howie Snizak and his wife Joan were there, Jerry and John Wood, Jack Holtz, Gene Reinhardt, Bill Proshek, Jimmy Knobloch, were all present and accounted for.

But the guys didn't stop there. Oh no. They had it set up for one of the local cops, Officer Bell, to come driving up in his patrol car—with the siren wailing, and the red lights on—to give me a ticket for fishing without a license! I didn't know this of course.

So the cop comes down, walks straight over to me, and says, "Mr. Hurley, what are you doing here? Let me see your *fishing license.*"

"I don't have a license, officer."

"Too bad. I'll have to give you a summons."

So he actually writes out a ticket, all dummied up of course, and hands it to me. "There goes my beer money. Thanks a lot." And everybody cracks up laughing.

We had a fish fry that afternoon, and I got my trout on opening day of the fishing season!


*ANN* Many of our friends were extremely good to us. Jerry and Georgia Wood, in particular. They were true friends. Even more than family. Your family you're stuck with. Friends you can pick. They were here constantly. Before, during, and after the transplant.

When John was released from Dover General, he still couldn't get out of his wheelchair. He had severe back pain while he was healing. So Jerry would come over by the hour. He's a fireman, and he'd have two and three days off at a time. I'm sure he had other things to do, but he'd come over and spend hours on end in the bedroom, entertaining John and me.

Or he'd come over and literally *carry* John up the stairs—force him to get out of the bedroom, put him in the wheelchair, and take him down to the boardwalk, to go fishing. Of course, John would be grumbling all the way.

So one day, Jerry says to me, "Ann, for a *fee,* how much is this lug insured for? We can get rid of this transplant! I'll release the brakes, and let him roll over, into the lake! And we can get rid of him if he's that much of a bastard!"

I said, "DO IT, JERRY! DO IT! DO IT!"

Toward the end of May, Jerry wanted to go over to the local tavern. He knew it was a favorite hangout of John's, and everybody wanted to see him. But John felt very awkward, very hesitant about being seen in there, in that condition.

Now Jerry is about 5'8"—and he says, "John, if we have to throw a blanket around you and *carry* you out *bodily,* we are leaving this house! You have *got* to get out of this house, and come over with me to the Tamarack!" And by God, he did it. He actually *carried* John to his car, put the wheelchair in the trunk, drove over to the Tamarack Inn, then carried John inside, *on his shoulders*! Everybody starts applauding. John was hanging on for dear life, and Jerry boosts him up to the bar and says, "Outta my way and clear the bar! I want to buy this guy a drink!"

Jerry had forced him to go. But that's what finally got John out of his shell. It was the one last push he needed.

Now, when the Hurley Fund was going, they used to have a contribution can in different places. And there was one still sitting in the Tamarack. So John sees it and gets a little embarrassed. He whispers to Jerry, "I don't want anybody shaking the can at me while I'm drinkin' a beer!"

"What?"

"Or thinking to himself, I'm putting money in there for that guy, and the son-of-a-bitch is out buying himself a beer with it."

So Jerry says, "Are you kidding? What the hell are you worried about *that* for? As a matter of fact, let's order a *double,* and drink it *outta the friggin' can!*"

*JOHN*   I guess I'm a bit of a local celebrity here in the township. Like when I go into the Tamarack. Everybody knows who I am. They always raise their glasses or nod at me when I come in. It's not that large a township. There's maybe four thousand residents, total. But you'd be surprised how many of the people you get to know.

So you'll be sitting there at the bar, and a guy'll come up to you and ask, "Hey John, do you ever think about having somebody else's heart inside you?"

I tell 'em, "Pal, it's *there.* Thank God it's there. And I'm glad it's still *working.* It's *great.* You know what I mean?"

"Lemme buy you a drink, John."


It was astounding the way the John Hurley Fund brought the township people closer together, when they found out I'd have to fly out to Stanford. I still can't get over it.

Shirley Berkowitz is a very special person. She did the majority of the work on the Fund, as the chairwoman. Volunteered her time for us. A remarkable woman. She was surprised too, how everyone pulled together to help us. Even the kids in school.

Like some friends of Janice organizing a "Friends of Janice" Bake Sale. It was amazing! They stuck flyers in the doors and mailboxes of all the people in the area, and in less than ninety minutes, 120 homemade cakes and pies were sold at the Andover A&P! Unbelievable! And all the money went to the John Hurley Fund. And this magician, "The Amazing Condor," gave two benefit magic shows over at the Forest Lakes Clubhouse. He was a big hit. A college kid. Name of Greg Shoun, of Greenbrook. And homemade "Crunch Bars" were sold at the high school, with all the proceeds going to the Fund. The Boy Scouts held this ten-mile "Walk-A-Thon" through the Washington Crossing State Park. They were sponsored by the Cranberry Lake Volunteer Fire Department, and the Scouts donated all the money to the Fund. And the cafeteria workers at the Lenape Valley High School made these special milkshakes (they called this a "Shake-A-Thon"!) and donated the money to the Fund. Everybody was drinking shakes!

Then there was a "Bike-A-Thon," where a bunch of kids rode twenty-eight miles on their bikes and donated everything their sponsors had contributed to the Fund. Janice rode in the Bike-A-Thon herself. She came home *covered* from head to toe with mud. Top to bottom. Almost couldn't see her face. But she said it was worth it. The mayor, Neil Gilling, he donated all the money that he would have used to buy Christmas cards and stamps that year, and instead of sending Christmas greetings to all his friends and neighbors, he donated this money to the Fund. The local Heart Association donated the at-home portable EKG machine that we're using now, so that we could make our own tests without having to go down to the doctor's office. Extremely necessary for us.

The Lenape Valley Women's Club raised money for us at a Benefit Tea Social. Did very nicely. Then there was a Benefit Dance at the Adam Todd Inn, with music and bands, and entertainment and comedians. And the Sheer Happiness Beauty Salon really did a terrific thing. They contributed all of their gross receipts from one whole day's business, on a John Hurley Benefit Sunday!

All together, the Fund helped us through some pretty rough times.

# 25

## The Second Acute Rejection

*JOHN*  I had my second acute rejection in July '75.

My voltage began dropping on the EKG. That's the sign of an imminent rejection. My average is up around 50 to 54. That week it dropped to 46, then to 40. I developed chills and fever. Then we knew. If there's a *five* percent drop, they become concerned. I called Dr. Kroner. He called Dr. Mason at Stanford, right away. They increased the Prednisone dosage from thirty milligrams up to a hundred milligrams. Then we waited.

Prednisone is an extremely powerful steroid, and it makes you very weak. It affects all your muscles. You start developing this hunger thing again. Your face becomes bloated. You start getting these blotches on your face. You start losing hair again. We hovered over the EKG. The next day, the voltage was up to 42. A good sign. The day after that, it was up to 44. The next day, 47. After that, it came steadily back. If it hadn't, they would've put me on a plane immediately, to Stanford, for massive therapy.

These rejections can occur at any time. Even years from now.

So I take my medications at 6:00 a.m., 9:00 a.m., 12:00 noon, 6:00 p.m., 9:00 p.m., and midnight. Every single day. *Religiously.* Miss *one* day, and it's *over*. I take fifty-five pills, four tablets, two packages of potassium, and two teaspoons of a stool softener. I keep these medicines in a large satchel with a padlock on it, to keep the children out. I carry the key in my wallet. Ann has a key, too. On the top of my dresser I have six vials, with the times marked on the caps indicating when I'm supposed to take each medication. Every morning I pour all of the required dosages into each vial. Then I'm set for the day. If we're going to be out for the day, I take whichever vials I'll need with me. If we go on vacation, I take the satchel along with us, and the EKG machine as well.

*ANN* It's very hard trying to keep the family intact. Trying to understand all of them, plus give them a lot of attention. Little John just accepts everything at this point. He's a baby. Too young to understand. But little Joan, she's very sensitive. Every time she passes our bedroom and the door is open, she tiptoes inside. And if John's napping, she'll go over to him and ask him, "Are you still alive, Daddy?" She's very attached to him. I think she's the closest to him of all.

When Janice's guinea pig, Herbie, died, Joanie went straight into the bedroom and told John, "You can't die today, Daddy."

He looks at her and says, "Why not, honey?"

"Because we already had one people in the family die today. *Herbie.*"

John was laughing so much, he had tears in his eyes. He said, "This poor kid!"

The other day we drove past a cemetery, and she saw a tombstone with a heart engraved on it. So she says, "I'm gonna buy one just like that, Mommy. For Daddy. When he dies."

John is driving the car when he hears this, and he does a doubletake! *"What* are you gonna do, Joanie?"

But everything is like this since John got his new heart. She stands over him in the morning to make sure he takes his medicine. Every morning! Six years old! She's a little withdrawn. Very quiet and shy. But adorable. A wonderful child. We're giving her tap, ballet, and acrobatic lessons. We bought her tap shoes and a little ballet outfit. I see her stretching a lot. Janice shows her how to stretch her legs, and by this morning, she was doing some tapping. She likes it.

Janice used to be a cheerleader. She's very outgoing in school. Then when she went to Lenape Valley High, she became a color guard. People have the highest regard for her. As a babysitter she was highly recommended. She was so much in demand *we* couldn't get her half the time. It's funny, though, that there's that contrast between her personality at home and the one she has in school. Almost like a dual personality.

When she graduated elementary school, they have a yearbook, and I never knew it until she graduated, but her friends all used to call her "Megaphone Mouth."

I couldn't believe this! I said, "Megaphone Mouth! You? You never *talk*!"

And she said, "Oh . . . I don't know where they got that from."

And I said, "You know where they got that from. You've got one of the biggest mouths in the school!"

Her friend Linda tells me, "You should see Janice in school. Boy, if she's two blocks away, you can hear her."

And I said, "I don't believe it." But she's come home hoarse after playing different games. I'd say, "Why? How did you lose your voice?"

"From screaming and yelling in the hallway."

"What the hell are you screaming and yelling in the hallway for?"

"We had to win the Spirit Stick, Momma."
"Oh. That explains it."
"Mom, the Spirit Stick is a very important thing to our class."
"I see."
"Whoever is loudest in the hallways wins the Spirit Stick for the next semester."
"Right, Janice."
And their class did win it. No doubt with the help of "Megaphone Mouth." It's a piece of *wood* painted red, white, and blue. Spirit Stick! I figured we got off lucky, her just being hoarse. There was a banana-eating contest as well!

*JOHN* I constantly find myself angry. Ann has become more independent. Much stronger. More outspoken than she's ever been. She calls a spade a spade, where before she'd be more polite about it—if she spoke up at all. I also think she's colder. It's probably because I'm not working. She's just come out of a sheltered type of a life, to the realization that sooner or later she's gonna be left alone. And she's gonna have to be making decisions. And this is something that for her is a complete change.

Until four years ago, I was the only domineering force in this house. I *ruled* this house. There was no question about it. She would *never* counter me, or interject herself. Now—if I chastise one of the kids (after maybe blowing my cool and doing it in temper), she'll come back at me and interject herself on behalf of the kids, in front of the kids. And that's something that goes against my grain. *Totally.* I have always said that if I'm wrong, regardless, don't correct me in front of the children. Let's talk about it afterwards. But *not* in front of the kids. I've always felt that way.

So I constantly find myself angry. All the time. At the frustration. Like not being able to physically exert myself. I can't even get out and mow the lawn.

My wife mows the lawn for me.

*ANN* I challenge him more. I no longer think that every time he says something, it's absolutely the law. Before, I would. I'd never *question* anything he said. I no longer feel he's the Lord and Master. Not because he's weak or he's had an illness. It's just from that time of him being sick, and me being by myself and having to take over for a while, I feel that I *am* capable. He had me believing I wasn't capable of doing most things, much less running a household. I was conditioned. Brainwashed! It was a discovery for me that I *can* take care of things. And I *am* independent. And I *can* take control. And I *can* run the house.

In a sense, I'm preparing for another life. Another kind of life. To be independent, and not have to depend on anyone else. If I had to depend on John like I did before, I wouldn't be able to function. People change when the conditions change. It used to be that John worked, brought in the money, and I was the wife and mother. That's all been turned around, although I can't support us yet.

But I *will.*

To be perfectly honest, it's been very distant between us since he's had his transplant. I don't know why. He doesn't confide much. He blames the medication. Sits and daydreams a lot, out the window. If you try to probe him and find out what's on his mind, he'll say, "Don't bother me now, Ann. It's nothing. Really."

But deep down, John is as afraid as anybody would be. He's broken down, emotionally, telling me he's frightened about what

I'm gonna have to face, and that I'm gonna be left to bear the brunt of our family's survival . . . and he hopes everything is gonna work out . . . and he's trying his best, financially. Sometimes . . . I can't bear to watch him. It's awful. His pain . . . As a man coming out of that tradition, he feels, as a *man,* very responsible to support his family. There must be a lot of guilt working when he knows he can't.

He's not as affectionate toward me as he used to be. I can honestly say that since his operation I've been extremely disappointed. I thought things would go back to even being affectionate sexually. But they haven't. John thinks that his sexuality has gotten better since the operation. But I don't really feel it has. He's very preoccupied with himself. Extremely preoccupied. I can't blame him though. He wasn't like that before. I don't know if it's the medication or not. He's cut the tranquilizers way down.

The medication definitely affects his mind. He's not as sharp as he used to be. I'll ask him a question and it takes him much longer to answer it than it did a few years ago. He used to be super-sharp.

"John? Are you listening to me? Is something wrong with your hearing?"

And he says, "I . . . don't . . . think . . . about it." He just stares. Maybe he's very depressed.

That's why in some ways I think he plays a game with himself about returning to work. Because he knows he's not as sharp as he was. He knows that if he went back to work it could never be the same for him. That must bother him very much.

He cried the last time someone called from Sea-Land. An old friend from Puerto Rico had been transferred up here, and the two of them spoke for an hour about all the different things they had done, and times when they worked together, and all the different promotions everybody's had. After he hung up, the tears just welled up in his eyes. Then he wept.

"Jeez . . . I wish I could go back to work. I really do. Oh *God* I really do." He said it to himself. I went over to him.

"It's only when you talk to someone from the company. It brings back all those memories. You're reminded of things."

"Ann . . . I really miss it."

"But John—."

"I really wanna go back."

"John . . . you *can't* go back. You're only kidding yourself. You can't go back to Sea-Land. You'd have to get a full medical OK. And you're extremely tired in the afternoons. You know that."

He's just living one big lie.

I don't think he knows or admits his truest feelings to himself. Because on top of thinking he might go back to Sea-Land one day, he'll say, "I'm ready for death."

And I say, "How can you be ready for death, John?"

"Because I don't care if I live or not. I've seen all that I want to see, I've gone to all the places I want to go. So I'm ready."

I flat out don't believe that, and I've told him so. I think it's human nature to want to live. And this guy's got a will to live like nobody has! If he wanted to die, why does he run to the doctor every time he starts going downhill? I asked him that one time. "If you're so ready for death, John, and you're gonna accept it because you're always so disgusted at yourself for always being sick, then how come you always call the ambulance? Why don't you just lie down on that bed and die?" He couldn't answer me there.

"Don't you think you really want to live?"

"No. I'm ready. I'm ready to die. I really am."

I can honestly say I never expected that much out of our married life. I expected children. But I never cared that much about money. That was John. I wanted more of a family man,

I guess. Being home more. Spending more time with the children.

I've told him that even though he keeps saying he's gonna die, and it'll be a traumatic experience for the kids, I think he's just plain copping out by keeping his distance from the kids. That eats at me, constantly. I think you can prepare them for his death. As young as they are. Kids have a way of understanding *everything*. But by keeping his emotional distance, he's cheating those kids out of the very warmth they'll need to carry them into the future. When he's no longer with them. He refuses to get close to them. Says he knows what he's doing. And not to interfere. Period. But he could prepare those children. You could sit down first, and speak to a doctor or a priest about how to prepare them. There are ways of preparing children. There are parents who are dying who've prepared their children. But John can't. Maybe he can't face that fact about his life. God knows it wouldn't be easy.

John is preoccupied with other things. Money. Security. Material things. Which are not as important to me. I really don't give a damn if I own this house. If I sold it tomorrow and moved into an apartment, I wouldn't care. I want the children to know John. That's what's really important to me. It's the most important thing, as far as I'm concerned. But John just doesn't feel that way. We argue constantly, around and around. He says his is a *man's* point of view.

He says, "Ann, reverse the situation. Put yourself in my position, and say *you* have a wife with two small children and a teen-ager—and as soon as you die (you're the husband), the disability payments from work *cease*. They *stop*. The money is *kaput*. There's no way in God's name your wife can *exist* without going out to work. And even then, a woman up here makes *peanuts*! Where is she gonna work? Where are *you* gonna work, Ann? Huh? Answer me that! There's no way in the *world* you'll be able to continue living in this house! Your whole life-style will change *completely!* Doesn't that bother you? Isn't it important for you to be able to maintain the standard of living you've become accustomed to? That's what I've worked for, my whole goddamn life, goddamn it!"

So we keep on arguing.

"You could still find time to get closer to the kids."

"No I can't! My financial responsibility just has me *thinking all the time!*"

"That's bull, John."

"No it's not, goddamn it! There's just no way of increasing my income, keeping up with the cost of living, and trying to figure out a way of getting ahead in this box we're in. And trying to educate the kids. Janice is closest to college age and she's almost ready. I'm definitely not gonna be around when the other two are college age. I'll never live that long. I know that. I know that. So I'm really taking it day by day. I can't get close to the kids now."

"Come on, John."

"No, I mean it. When I get up in the morning and look outside the sliding glass doors, *which I paid for,* by the way, I'm thankful that I'm able to look outside at all."

"But that's my point!"

"What is?"

"The little ones are *not* going to know their father."

"That's right!"

"And whether you want to admit it or not, John, you can't *bear* to look at the kids and try to prepare them for the fact that you may not *be* here next week, or next month—which you keep saying doesn't really bother you because you're ready for it."

"That's not true!"

"Even if you *were* ready for it, which I seriously doubt, the question is, are *they*?"

"I don't know what you mean."

"Have you prepared *them* for it? For your death? God knows it wouldn't be easy! But if we can try and prepare them to be better children, and I don't mean money, then we should be doing all we can right now for that part of it. *Sure* I'm worried about how I'm going to support the kids! But we don't have to have the best of *everything,* as long as they have their father's *companionship,* and I have, for as long as we possibly can! And not you just sitting and figuring out *budgets*—to preoccupy yourself. I think it's more of a cop-out! I really do."

# 26

## A New Life

**JOHN**  I went back to college, five mornings a week. Taking a full twelve credits. They extended the GI benefits. I'm taking management, finance, advanced accounting, and an English appreciation course. I'm the oldest one in the class. County College of Morris.

I enjoy going back to school. A lot more than when I first went as a youngster. Now I appreciate it. I only wish I was young and able to swing with some of those chicks going around braless! Ann says, "So *that's* why you like going back to school. Ah *hah*!" The first time I went to that school, and this was summertime, and it was hot as hell down there, and you see these golden girls walking around; they don't leave *anything* to the imagination. I said to Ann, "Boy! This is gonna be some summer session! Wow-wow!" Sometimes I envy this younger generation. For being so free and open about sex. But on the other hand, like a friend of mine once said, "If it isn't *dirty,* you're not doing it right!"

The other morning I was going out to school. It was 8:00 a.m. and, so help me, here's this big *raccoon* down at the end of the sundeck! It was enormous! Looking right at me! I know they're nocturnal creatures, and when you see one during the day, it could be sick—and dangerous. And he was blocking my path to the car. So I call Ann out. "Look at that son-of-a-gun sitting there."

And it starts coming toward me. So I says, "Ann. Get me a rock." So she gets a rock and I throw it at it. Nothing. Keeps walking toward me. So I grab the broom and throw the broom at it. The damn thing walks right over the broom without batting an eyelash and keeps on coming after me. Stalking me.

So we run into the house, and the 'coon is sitting right in front of the back door. Ann gets a potato and throws it out the window—and the 'coon goes for it. Then she says, "Now hurry up and get to school!"

So I sneak out the front door, and as I'm heading for the car, with my briefcase and my brown bag lunch, and *The Wall Street Journal* under my arm, the son-of-a-bitch turns around—looks up at me—and starts racing after me! I'm running like a bastard, and he's right behind me, nipping at my heels, and I just make it into the car when he jumps up on the door and is staring at me through the window! Holding himself up by his claws! Looking at me with his beady little eyes! He would've jumped onto the front seat with me!

Now—I'm not afraid of raccoons, per se. But if it was rabid or something, and he managed to even *scratch* me, forget it. I'm dead. Because I'm immunosuppressed. There's nothing they could do for me. So I backed the car out of the driveway and peeled out.

Ann told me that the 'coon came back later, with a friend, and they finished the potato.

*ANN*  Since our loss of income, we've been forced to find every possible way to economize. Before John's heart attack, we only bought the finest cuts of meat, at the butcher, and never mind how much it cost. It had to be the best. I hardly ever bothered to look at the receipt. But things have changed.

This is farm country up here. Thank God. The farmers grow eggplant, tomatoes, corn, string beans, and green peppers. In the summertime, when beefsteak tomatoes are out, you get up to 8 pounds for a dollar. And you pick your own. And peppers, we buy a whole bushel for $3.50. Maybe 65 peppers. They'll last us through the whole season. Corn, if you pick your own, you can get 140 ears for $5.00. You clean them, boil them for two to three minutes, and freeze them. That's it. A lot of farmers raise cattle up here. So we can go out and buy a whole steer and take it to the local slaughterhouse. We buy the hindquarter for the sirloin steaks, roasts, and chopped meat. The best cuts are from the hindquarter. We get them wrapped, marked, and fast-frozen. You might spend $175.00, but this will last us the whole winter! Especially if you throw in a little chicken now and then. And John is fishing during the summer so we have trout frozen also.

The large freezer we bought was a good investment. Up at the A&P or Shop-Rite, if they have a sale, I'll go that week, if we have the extra money, and I'll buy a large quantity of whatever's on sale. Then I'll freeze it. If it's chickens, I'll buy maybe 25 of them. All year, it's a lot less for food if you keep watching for the "specials." We save hundreds of dollars.

John hunts, also, so we have venison and pheasant that the great white explorer bags himself. I can't bring myself to eat anything John kills. Janice can, though. She loves venison. I wouldn't touch a piece of it. I cook it, smell it, and gag.

**JOHN** There are restrictions as far as salt and cholesterol are concerned. When I first had the heart attack, I was taken off salt altogether. That's four years now. So I use that imitation salt. I find no difference whatsoever. With the cholesterol, there are certain foods I *do* miss. Like pork chops. And ham. I haven't had ham *at all*. I've had broiled pork chops *twice,* in four years.

As far as calories go, I'm careful. I make sure to eat less than they allow me to, with the only exception being liquor. We're just not sure how many calories are in liquor. And I haven't done *anything* to find out, either! In California, they said I could have two ounces of booze a day. Protect me, oh Lord!

I'm allowed to have four ounces of cooked meat a day. Six fruits. I like vegetables and I like salads, so I fill up on those a lot. Maybe once a month I'll have an egg. *One* egg. I used to eat them at least three times a week. Now I eat these egg substitutes, and these cholesterol-free soy-protein sausage patties. I enjoy them. It's sometimes hard to tell the difference, really. Especially when you're holding your nose!

TV dinners are the worst thing you can have. They have so much salt and preservatives in them. They tell you to beware these prepared foods and canned vegetables, because of the added salt. Sugar is off limits, too. Because of the Prednisone. It leaves you prone to becoming a diabetic. Can set in overnight.

I haven't had a frankfurter in four years. They tell you that franks are one of the worst things *anyone* can eat. Not just heart patients. They're made out of nothing but fats, salts, preservatives, and the lowest gristle and grades of meat possibly imaginable. Same with cold cuts. There are signs up at Stanford which actually say, "BE GOOD TO YOUR HEART. DON'T EAT FRANKFURTERS, COLD CUTS, LIVER, SHELLFISH, OR SAUSAGE MEATS."

I love *matzohs*. Love 'em. They have no salt. All it is is flour and water. I could sit down and eat a whole box of matzohs. I get them all the time. Garlic flavored. Onion flavored. Regular. My sideburns haven't been getting any longer, though! I've checked! I'm allowed to have some starch. Like bread, potatoes, or macaroni. And when I'm planning to have spaghetti for dinner, I drop the other starches from that day's diet. I've cut back a *lot* with Italian food.

*ANN* John had spaghetti the other night. A big bowl of it. A *vegetable bowl* full! *Marrone!* And an *entire* loaf of Italian bread. With garlic and oil on it. With salad on the side. He overdoes it some nights. He finished it all and asked for more! If you say, "No more, John," he really gets nasty. Like an animal.

"Goddamn it! I'll tell *you* when I've had enough! Don't stand there, looking over my shoulder and supervising what I eat, for crissakes!"

Then after he's finished, he'll say, "Jeez, I shouldn't have had that much. Now I went and blew my whole diet."

"Then why did you do it? You knew you shouldn't be eating that much."

"I know. But I could eat a *pound* of spaghetti myself. I really could."

"Could? Could? You just *did.*"

He makes his own sauce, too. Lets it simmer the whole day. From morning till night. Hovers over it, like a mad scientist, checking it hourly, adding a little bit of this spice and a little bit of these herbs, and always stirring gently. Lovingly. Like a master chef. He always makes so much that there's a quart left over, and when that happens, he fills a soup bowl with it, then takes half a loaf of Italian bread, and he and Janice polish it off together. He shouldn't. But he does.

The other day, we were in a luncheonette, and we saw a sign, "TODAY'S SPECIAL: HOT CHILI." I looked at him, he looked at me, and sure enough, he ordered it. The sweat was pouring off him as he ate it. The waitress, seeing him perspire like a fountain, comes over and says, "Is it *that* hot?" John says, "No. But could you turn the air conditioning up just a little bit higher, please?" You see, the chili wasn't "hot" enough for him. He added a teaspoonful of pepper to it, besides!

I get him home and I said, "Hurley, you sure you needed that chili?"

And he says, "Look Ann, I'm making the best of this diet. I'm making it livable! Can't you understand that? I'm a *human being*! I can't just eat salads twenty-four hours a day! I'm not a goddamn rabbit, for crissakes!"

"I know John, but look—."

"Look nothing. My breakfast is a slice of white toast, glass of orange juice which I have my medicine in, and two cups of tea. Lunch I'll have a salad with a glass of milk. At dinner I might have a baked potato and a steak. I can only have red meat three times a week! The rest has to be fish and chicken because they're low in cholesterol. I have my vodka and tonics. And that's *it*! That's bloody *it*! So I've *gotta* be able to cheat now and then! You can understand that, can't you, Ann?"


*JOHN* Today, if you were to ask me, "John, what is life all about?" I'd have to say, "Phil, right now, life is to *live. L-I-V-E.*" I think that after you've gone through what I've gone through, you change your outlook. Your life-style is changed *for you.* And that's an understatement! But who knows? Maybe tomorrow they'll come up with an artificial heart. Maybe nuclear-powered!

And M. I. T. has a research program for preserving (by freezing) vital organs for later transplantation. The possibilities are exciting.

I live with a certain degree of hope. That they will find something that will increase the longevity. It's possible. It's very possible. Hopefully, they will. Dr. Shumway told me they've got people working on finding substitutes for the steroids I'm on. But I'm realistic. It may not be in my time. I have no doubt, though, whatsoever, that the breakthrough will occur, sometime in the future.

Ann gives me an EKG test twice a week, to detect any voltage drops. We've got the machine, a little portable unit not much bigger than a typewriter, set up on my nightstand, next to the bed. A couple of weeks ago the readings were *alarmingly* low. *So* low I started to sweat. Ann became hysterical. Then I remembered hearing that any drop on the power line as generated by the power company could show up that way on my readings. It was the only explanation. Either that or I was ready to meet my Maker. So I called the billing office over at Jersey Power and Light Company, and I explained to them that I was a heart transplant and I wanted to know if there was a power reduction at the time I was taking my EKG. They gave me the name of the person to contact, who was over in Lake Hopatcong. I explained the situation to him and he checked all his records, and even gave me his home phone number to call in the event it happened again. This particular time, after checking through all his records, he found out that sure enough, thank the Lord, there *had* been a dip in their generated power, which accounted for the low readings.

As part of my periodic checkups, I have to go down to the hospital to take a stress test. They hook you up to an EKG machine and monitor your blood pressure and pulse rate. And they have you ride a bicycle that's held stationary in place. They set it at different speeds and pressures, with a brake on the wheels, for drag, so it gets harder and harder to peddle. Then they put you through your paces and record everything. Next, they put you on a treadmill, and speed you up so you're almost in a trot. Extremely fast walking motions and elevations, as if you were jogging up a hill, so they can tell how your heart is operating under these stress conditions. I still have to wear my mask when I enter the hospital for these tests. The Lone Ranger rides again!

I'll never know it if I have another heart attack, because certain nerves in my chest have been severed. I won't feel the chest pain that another person might feel. I will feel "hot flashes," and an increased pulse rate, especially around the veins in the neck. But I'm gonna fight like hell. I'll tell you that right now. Right down to the last. I'm not gonna give up and just let it wash over me. Not by any means. No sir. If I have a choice, I'm gonna fight *right down to the tooth and nail of it.*

I believe in God. And I believe deep down in a hereafter. Because I think everybody has to have a belief. Everybody has to have someone to look up at every once in a while, to pray to, to have confidence in, or talk to. You know . . . sometimes you can't talk to people. So I say my prayers silently to myself. Every night.

But I don't believe in asking God for something for *myself.* I'm thankful for what I *receive.* I don't believe He's the miracle man that you can ask favors of. Especially materialistic things. Definitely not. If someone were sick, you might ask, "Please watch over him." Or something like that. But even at that point I wouldn't beg for favors. Never. I'd say, "Thank you for letting Ann's father live. Thank you for sparing my father's eyesight. That it's not getting any worse." But even through my illness, I've never asked for help in seeing myself through it. Never.

Asking for something is strange for me. Maybe that's a hangup of mine. Let's say I need a thousand dollars tomorrow, I wouldn't ask anyone for it. I'd find a way of getting it by doing it on my own. Or not get it at all. Period.

I don't associate my medical problems with God. It has to do with the fact that everybody on this earth has a date on 'em. And when that date comes, whether you die of a heart attack, or you're walking in the street and just trip over a *toy,* if your time has come, it's come. And that's it. It's Destiny.

I'd like to be buried above ground. In a mausoleum made out of Belgian block marble. A magnificent tomb. I've already discussed it with some buddies of mine who are masons, that that's what I want. They've told me that when the time comes, they'll build it for me whenever it becomes necessary.

I took Ann over to the cemetery in Stanhope. It's only fifteen minutes from the house by car. And I showed her the mausoleum I liked. Gave her a tour of the place. The lawns. The gardens.

She gets tears in her eyes. "You must be kidding."

"I'm not kidding, Ann. This is where I'd like to be buried. I'm serious about this. I think these things should be planned for before you die. I'm in a position to *know* I'm gonna be dying, sooner rather than later. And I know *where.* So I'm in a position to go around and say what I want—about where I'm gonna be buried. I don't think that's being unreasonable. Do you, Ann?"

So all she does is look at me, straight in the eye. "Tell you what, John. *Sue me!*"

# 27

## Champagne

*JOHN* November 16, 1975, marked one year since the transplant. My first anniversary. And the following week was Thanksgiving. As it happened, my birthday fell on Thanksgiving Day. November 27th. I turned forty.

We rented a villa up in Pennsylvania. Spent a week up there, just to relax. The villa itself was beautifully modern, really plush, with wall-to-wall carpeting, spacious rooms, a complete kitchen, all-electric, featuring a GE trash compactor, dishwasher, refrigerator-freezer combination, a washer, a dryer, a self-cleaning stove, all utensils, pots and pans, glasses, and central air conditioning.

Janice wasn't able to be with us the whole time, because she had to work at the A&P and they wouldn't give her all that time off. So I drove in on Wednesday and picked her up, so she could be with us through the rest of the week. We spent a nice, quiet Thanksgiving and birthday celebration. Just our family. Together.

The kids had plenty to keep them occupied. Swimming in the indoor pool, and playing on the swings and monkeybars in the playground. Could go for hours and hours. They have six tennis courts up there, the indoor heated pool, two outside pools, an arts-and-crafts room for children, a disco lounge, a bar, a country club room, a driving range, and a twenty-seven-hole golf course. Ann and I are getting pretty good with our golf lessons, and the weather was very mild. We shot some darn good rounds. I surprised myself. Shot nine holes. Then we went out with Janice to watch the Swiss ski instructor make some practice runs on the ski slopes. Janice had been dying to see him work out. He was sensational. Spectacular.

Later that afternoon—a funny thing—stepping into the sauna they have up there, with my towel wrapped around me, I suddenly thought of my old pal, Al Weinstein. And the Navy. And the "baths." As I entered the place, and I'm trying to see through all the mist, I see this guy in there, I see this guy looking very much the way Weinstein might look today, all these years later. Very similar face and features. For a second, I couldn't believe my eyes. I must have stared at the guy for a full minute. Then I went over to him.

"Your name wouldn't be Weinstein, would it?"

"Sorry. No."

"Oh. It's just that you look like someone I used to be friends with."

It's funny. The things you think of. At the oddest times.

That night, the waitress brought a large chocolate-cream birthday cake with forty candles on it. Ann and the kids sang "Happy Birthday" to me, then applauded. Everybody at the surrounding tables looked over at us and smiled. I made my wish. I said it to myself. That God should protect my family after

I'm gone. After I finished, the kids blew out all the candles.

When we got back to the villa, Ann put the kids to bed. Janice had a book she was reading, so she stayed in with the little ones. For the moment, I was alone. Ann was telling the kids what they'd be doing tomorrow. Little Joan wanted to ride on a horse, and I could hear Ann telling her that it was too cold for horses, but she could ride on a horse in the summer.

I lit a fire. Put newspaper under the pine logs in the fireplace and got it going real good. Then I got out the glasses and poured myself some champagne. I looked around the room. All natural woods on the floor, walls, and ceilings, and this cane-and-wicker furniture. And the big brick fireplace. I thought about the holidays.

The Christmas and Thanksgiving holidays have always been cherished by us. It's a family type of a thing, where all of us get together. Real enjoyable days. Everybody usually winds up in Norene's house. She doesn't necessarily plan on having everybody, but it always works out that way, at the last minute. Ann has four sisters and two brothers, and they all have three and four children apiece, and there are nieces that are grown, and *they* have children. I remember a couple of years ago, when we all got together for Thanksgiving. Either Ann or Norene cooked three twenty-pound turkeys! What an electric bill! And we had champagne, and all the trimmings, and everybody had one hell of a mellow time. It was a beautiful evening. We all told jokes and stories, and the kids were running around making a mess and bumping into everything. Little John wound up with a bowl of cole slaw on his head. We still don't know how that happened! And I remember seeing Ann's parents dancing together. Somebody had put some nice music on. And we both saw her father giving her mother a kiss on the cheek. They really looked romantic. Happy.

Just then I felt a hand on my shoulder. I looked up, and it was Ann. I was so busy looking into the fire that I hadn't heard her come into the room.

"So how come my glass is empty?"

"I didn't want it to go flat."

"Right."

"Here. I'll pour you some now."

I filled her glass and refilled mine. She looked over toward the kids' room.

"All tucked. Joanie wants a horse."

"She wants to ride a horse?"

"No. She wants us to *buy* her a horse."

"Oh. I see."

We were sitting down on a very comfortable old couch. And all of a sudden we looked at each other and realized something about each other. We both got the same idea at the same time. We clinked our champagne glasses together. It was a meaningful moment for the two of us. Something special.

I said, "You know something, babe? I really love you."

"I love you too, John."

Then I looked into her eyes and raised my glass to her once again.

"You know something, Ann? I just thought of something."

"Yeah?"

"I *just* realized something about the two of us."

"What's that, John?"

"You know why we're still together?"

"Say what?"

"Even after everything?"

"I'll bite."

"Because neither one of us ever had the *balls* to walk out the door *first*!"

And you know how true that is? How true that really is? Most people stay together because they don't have the *courage* to leave! Especially if there are children. It's harder to leave than to stay! Leaving presents more problems than staying! That's some testimonial to marriage! But I know that Ann and I could never have put up with all that's happened to us if we didn't love each other. And that's it right there, pal. Tremendous!

*Author's Note*

John Hurley died on Monday, November 15, 1976, of an infection complicated by his immunosuppressive drug therapy. The autopsy revealed no evidence whatever of transplant rejection.

To:

Dr. Richard S. Kroner, who saved my life.

Dr. Norman E. Shumway, and the transplant team at Stanford University Medical Center, for extending it.

Father John Hester, for his spiritual guidance and support. And much, much more.

Our family, friends, and neighbors, for their unstinting generosity and prayers.

My friends, associates, and fellow-employees of Sea-Land Service throughout the world, for their many kindnesses.

The Roxbury Medical Center personnel who donated their lunch hours to take X-rays, blood tests, and EKGs of me without charge.

The family of the donor, whose identity we still do not know, whose gift quite literally made it possible for me to continue.

And to our three wonderful children.

This book is lovingly dedicated to you all.

JOHN and ANN HURLEY

# *Acknowledgments*

I should like to express my gratitude to my editor, Patricia Irving, for her patience, understanding, and skill.

I also wish to thank Ralph Rosenblum, Maureen Rolla, Professor Jesse J. Dossick, Erna Kolbert, Joanna Lee Harbert, Michael Harbert, Eileen Ain, Henry Viola, Ruth Smerechniak, Stephen Elliot Dossick, Stephen Gillers, and my agent, Peter L. Skolnik, for help generously given in a variety of ways.